Colour Atlas of
Paediatric Haematology

Colour Atlas of
Paediatric Haematology

Second Edition

Ian M. Hann MD, MRCP, MRCPath.
Brian D. Lake PhD., FRCPath.
Jon Pritchard FRCP

The Hospital for Sick Children, Great Ormond Street, London

and

John Lilleyman FRCP, FRCPath.

The Childrens Hospital, Sheffield

Oxford   New York   Toronto   Melbourne
OXFORD UNIVERSITY PRESS
1990

Oxford University Press, Walton Street, Oxford OX2 6DP
Oxford New York Toronto
Delhi Bombay Calcutta Madras Karachi
Petaling Jaya Singapore Hong Kong Tokyo
Nairobi Dar es Salaam Cape Town
Melbourne Auckland
and associated companies in
Berlin Ibadan

Oxford is a trade mark of Oxford University Press

Published in the United States
by Oxford University Press, New York

© *Oxford University Press 1990*

British Library Cataloguing in Publication Data
Colour atlas of paediatric haematology.—2nd ed.
1. Children. Blood. Diseases
I. Hann, Ian M.
618.92'15
ISBN 0-19-261893-8

Library of Congress Cataloging in Publication Data
Colour atlas of paediatric haematology/Ian M. Hann . . . [et al.].—2nd ed.
Bibliography Includes index.
1. Pediatric hematology—Atlases. I. Hann, Ian M.
[DNLM: 1. Hematologic Diseases—in infancy & childhood—atlases.
WS17 C719]
RJ411.C64   1989   618.92'15—dc20   89-9347
ISBN 0-19-261893-8

Typeset, Printed and Bound in Hong Kong

Foreword to the first edition

by

David Weatherall

Nuffield Professor of Clinical Medicine,
University of Oxford

There must be few 'adult haematologists' who have not gazed in gloomy despair at a blood film from a newborn infant and speculated uneasily on whether the bizarre morphological changes of the red cells were within normal limits. Certainly, I have spent a few sleepless nights over wild white cell changes in the blood of young children with viral illnesses, wondering if I was seeing an unusual form of leukaemia or whether it was just a reflection of the perversity of childhood to react to infection in this way. Indeed, it is sobering to reflect that the majority of haematologists who look at blood films or bone marrows of infants or young children have had little or no training in paediatrics. In many countries, and Great Britain is no exception, paediatric haematology is the Cinderella of the paediatric sub-specialities. Most paediatricians, like general physicians, are unable to find their way round a blood film or marrow and are totally reliant on their laboratory colleagues, often only experienced in adult blood diseases, for assessing the significance of the haematological findings in sick children. For this reason the authors of this atlas have done a particularly valuable job in bringing together a representative series of pictures of the blood and marrow, both from normal infants and children and from those with haematological disorders peculiar to childhood. I imagine that this book will become a constant companion to haematologists who are called on occasionally to look at the blood or marrow of sick children. At least they will be reassured to see that laboratory artefacts seem to be the same in adult and paediatric practice.

The scope of paediatric haematology has increased immensely over the last few years. It is now possible to obtain blood samples early in fetal life, many new genetic disorders of the blood cells have been defined, the sub-classification of the acute leukaemias has assumed importance in both prognosis and treatment, and a frighteningly complex series of storage disorders have been identified, many of which may present for the first time to the haematologist. With the rapid movement of people round the world paediatric haematologists are often presented with bizarre parasites in the blood, and genetic diseases like the haemoglobinopathies, which used to be so rare in North European countries, are now being seen with increasing frequency in immigrant populations. All these new developments are reflected in this atlas.

Paediatric haematology has made a major contribution to the more fundamental aspects of haematological research over the last few years. While in the age of monoclonal antibodies and DNA sequencing it might seem rather old-hat to produce a new atlas of blood morphology, it should be remembered that the application of these new and highly sophisticated techniques is useless unless there has been an accurate morphological diagnosis of the condition being studied. Hence I suspect that this book will also find its way into departments who are working on fundamental haematological research.

Apart from being an acute reminder of increasing age, it is a particular pleasure to be invited to write a foreword to a book in which two of the authors are one's former research fellows or house staff; those involved in medical education need constantly reassuring that it is very difficult permanently to damage the young. I am certain that this atlas will fill an important gap for clinicians and research workers in both developed and developing countries and I wish this first edition, and those that will undoubtedly follow, much success. It is particularly satisfying to see a book of this type coming from the Haematology Department at Great Ormond Street where so much has been done to try to push forward a subject which has, with the exception of one or two centres, been rather neglected in this country.

Preface to second edition

We blushingly received a number of complimentary remarks after publication of the first edition of this Atlas, but also became aware of some errors and omissions, several of them pointed out by readers, reviewers, or colleagues. Besides adding, in the second edition, a good deal of new material, especially to the sections dealing with acute leukaemia, perinatal disorders, and storage disorders, we have attended to those deficiencies. The result, we think, is a better, more comprehensive Atlas. John Lilleyman's contribution has been much appreciated by the other three authors —his organized mind and special experience have added crispness and breadth.

We thank Sonia Taylor and Marie Elliott for patient secretarial help, and Professor Sir David Weatherall for support and encouragement.

London   I.M.H. B.D.L.
May 1989   J.L. J.P.

Preface to first edition

For those accustomed to the microscopic appearances of blood and bone marrow films of adults, the interpretation of paediatric material can sometimes present problems. Marked leucocytosis or leuco-erythroblastosis in a neonate or the blood or bone marrow lymphocytosis of later infancy might, for instance, suggest serious infection or even leukaemia to the microscopist unfamiliar with these 'normal' appearances. In addition, the spectrum of disorders presenting to a paediatric haematology laboratory only overlaps that seen in its adult counterpart. Some disorders (e.g. chronic lymphatic leukaemia and myelofibrosis) are exceptional in childhood, whilst others (e.g. neuroblastoma and many storage disorders) are almost exclusive to it; in addition, some cytological appearances (e.g. megaloblastic bone marrow) are likely to have a quite different patho-physiological basis than in adults.

In this Atlas, introduced by a section on 'normal' appearances, we have tried to illustrate most of the haematological disorders—both common and uncommon—that might be encountered by haematologists and technical staff. Because haematologists are increasingly being asked to help in their interpretation, we have included a section on the cytology of the more common of the 'solid' childhood malignancies in body fluids and in lymph node touch preparations. Marrow trephine biopsies and electron microscopic appearances are included where they make a significant contribution to diagnosis. Finally, and because of important recent refinements in cytochemical diagnostic techniques, we have devoted a section to storage disorders.

Our hope and intention is that this atlas will be an *aide-memoire* for both haematologists and technical staff, particularly those working in an adult context, to the differential diagnosis of haematological disorders seen in infancy and childhood. We have therefore tried to index and cross-index all of the illustrations as thoroughly as possible. On the other hand, we have felt that an exhaustive bibliography is superfluous to our purpose and have limited ourselves to providing a few key references to sources of information about individual conditions. For those interested in our own cytochemical techniques we have included references to methods for the stains currently used in our laboratories.

We hope that the atlas will be of help and interest to those dealing with children's disease.

September 1982

I. M. H.   A. R.
B. D. L.   J. P.

Acknowledgements

Many individuals contributed materials for use in the atlas. We are very grateful to the following colleagues within the Hospital for Sick Children, Great Ormond Street, London: Mr Robert Brock; Professor Judith Chessells; Professor Roger Hardisty; Dr J. Kemshead; Dr Elizabeth Letsky; Dr Marian Malone; Mr Stephen Mills; Dr Nick Rapson. We are also indebted to colleagues in other institutions for their contributions: Mrs Lesley Bloom BSc, FIMLS (Ravenscourt Laboratories); Miss Julie Cameron FIMLS and Mr David Wheeler FIMLS, MIBiol. (Royal Berkshire Hospital); Dr Ken Clark (Guy's Hospital); Dr David Evans (Royal Manchester Children's Hospital); Dr Ted Gordon-Smith and Dr S. M. Lewis (Hammersmith Hospital); Dr R. Goudsmit (Academisch Ziekenhuis, Amsterdam); Professor Ralph Hendrickse (Liverpool); Professor A. V. Hoffbrand (Royal Free Hospital); Dr Bernadette Modell (University College Hospital); also Dr M. C. Galvin (Pinderfields Hospital), Mr D. Barnett and Mrs J. Britton (Sheffield).

Contents

Abbreviations

ALL	acute lymphoblastic leukaemia
AML	acute myeloblastic leukaemia
ANA	antinuclear antibody
C-ALL	common acute lymphoblastic leukaemia antigen
CDA	congenital dyserythropoietic anaemia
CGL	chronic granulocytic leukaemia
CMV	cytomegalovirus
CNS	central nervous system
CSF	cerebrospinal fluid
DIC	disseminated intravascular coagulation
DNA	deoxyribonucleic acid
EB	Epstein–Barr (virus)
EDTA	ethylenediaminetetraacetic acid (anticoagulant)
HE	haematoxylin and eosin (stain)
Hb	haemoglobin
Hb F	fetal haemoglobin
Hb H	haemoglobin H
HDN	haemolytic disease of the newborn
HEMPAS	hereditary erythroblast multinuclearity with positive acid serum lysis test (CDA type II)
ITP	idiopathic thrombocytopenic purpura
LE	lupus erythematosus
LNTP	lymph node touch preparation
MGG	May–Grünwald–Giemsa (stain)*
MPS	mucopolysaccharidosis
NAP	neutrophil alkaline phosphatase
NBT	nitro blue tetrazolium
PAS	periodic acid Schiff (stain)
RAEB	refractory anaemia with excess of blasts
RAEB(T)	refractory anaemia with excess of blasts in transformation
T-ALL	acute leukaemia derived from T-lymphoblasts
TP	touch preparation
VMA	vanilylmandelic acid

* Staining is with MGG unless otherwise stated. Details of magnification have only been included where they are of real significance.

1
Normal appearances

1.1. **Early pronormoblast** (Arrow)
Bone marrow
This plate shows a large basophilic normoblast. Nucleoli are present. The cytoplasm is intensely basophilic because of its high RNA content.

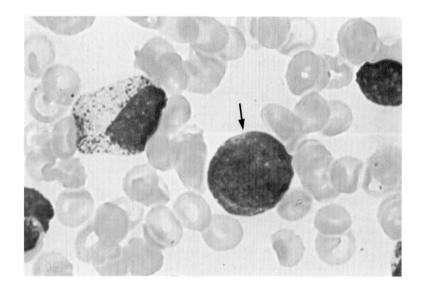

1.2. **Early basophilic normoblast** (Arrow)
Bone marrow
This cell has slightly less RNA than 1.1; haemoglobin synthesis has started so the basophilia is less intense than in 1.1. A myelocyte, a band (stab) cell, and a lymphocyte are also present.

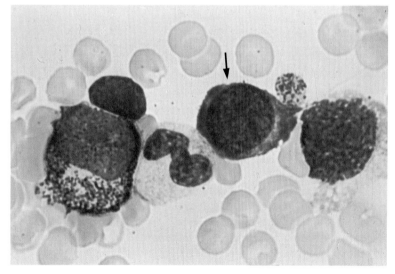

1.3. Developing normoblasts
Bone marrow

This plate shows an intermediate (polychromatic) and a late orthochromatic normoblast. The polychromasia of the intermediate normoblast (below) is a result of its lesser RNA and greater haemoglobin content than that of earlier forms. The orthochromia in the later cell (above) is the result of its increasing haemoglobin content so that the cell takes up the acidophilic component of MGG stain.

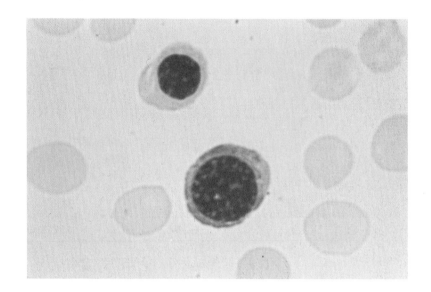

1.4. Late normoblast
Bone marrow

This small well-haemoglobinized normoblast (arrowed) and another cell with disintegrating nucleus represent the last stages of normoblast development. A myelocyte is also present.

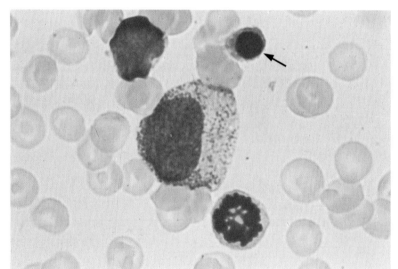

1.5. Promyelocyte
This is the first differentiated form of developing granulocytes. Nucleoli are visible and most of the granules are the primary azurophilic type. Some 1 per cent of normal marrow cells are promyelocytes.

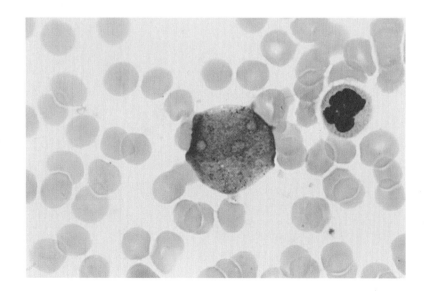

1.6. Developing granulocytes (1)

Four stages of maturation can be seen in this frame; promyelocyte (pm), myelocyte (m), metamyelocyte (mm), and mature neutrophil (n). Two erythroblasts (eb) are also present.

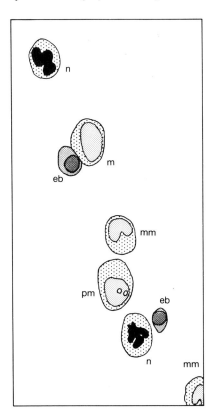
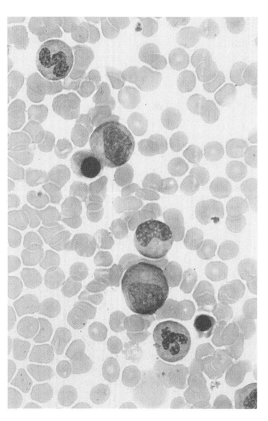

1.7. Developing granulocytes (2)

Further variants of maturing granulocytes identified as in 1.6.

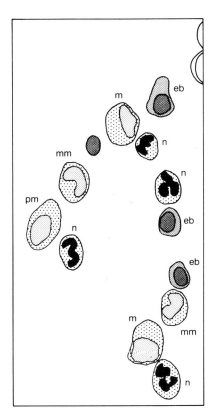
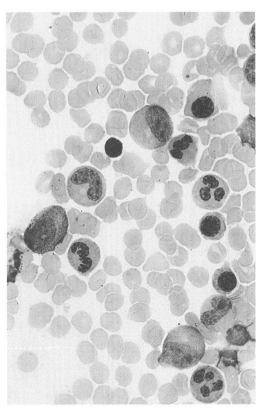

1.8. Band or stab cell
Blood

This cell is the intermediate precursor of the mature polymorph—neutrophil in this instance. The nucleus is crescentic rather than lobed. These early forms are seen in increased numbers in the blood in response to infection.

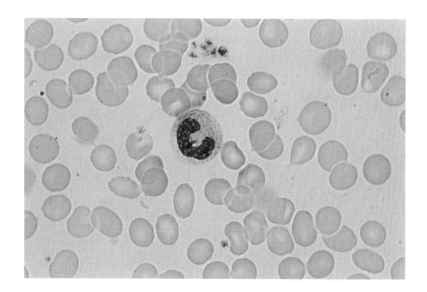

1.9. Neutrophil polymorph
Blood

The mature granulocyte usually has a three- to four-lobed nucleus. The nuclear chromatin is clumped and there are no nucleoli. Nuclear lobes are reduced in infection (shift to the left) and the Pelger—Hüet anomaly (see 4.3). Increased lobulation is present in megaloblastic anaemia (see 3.6, 3.7 and 3.8).

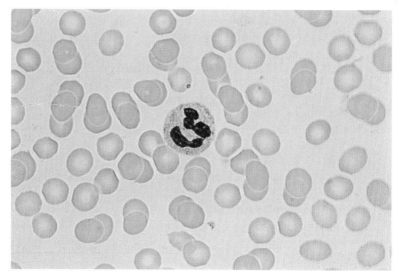

1.10. Eosinophil
Blood film
Eosinophils have orange granules on Romanowsky stains. Typically they are bilobed. They do not normally exceed 0.4 $\times$ 10^9/l. They are increased in allergy, atopy, in response to invasive parasites, drugs, and Hodgkin's disease. Rare primary eosinophilias occur, both benign and malignant.

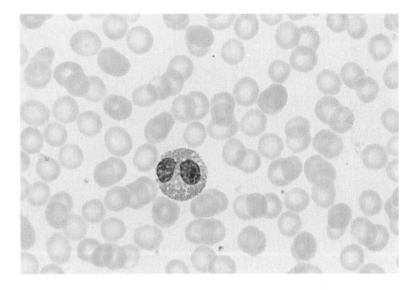

1.11. Basophil
Blood film
Basophils are the least common granulocytes and do not normally exceed 0.1 $\times$ 10^9/l. They are easily recognized. They may be elevated in hypothyroidism or chickenpox, but are most commonly seen in increased numbers in myeloproliferative disorders.

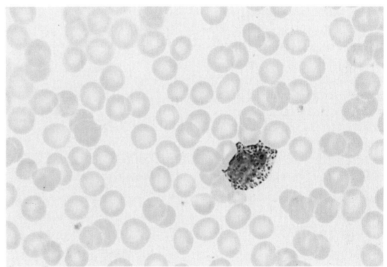

1.12. Monocytes
Blood film
Monocytes are derived from a precursor cell common to granulocytes. They typically have irregular nuclei and pale blue cytoplasm on Romanowsky staining. They do not normally exceed 0.8 $\times$ 10^9/l. Vacuoles and a few azurophil granules are sometimes evident. They increase in some chronic bacterial infections, infestations, virus infections, and autoimmune inflammatory disorders.

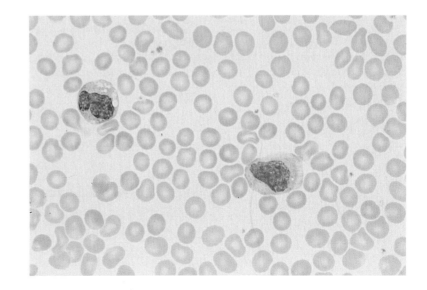

1.13. Mature lymphocyte
Blood film

A normal small, mature lymphocyte with scanty cytoplasm is shown. The blood lymphocyte count varies with age (see appendix of normal values) and may also be increased in infections (see lymphocyte disorders).

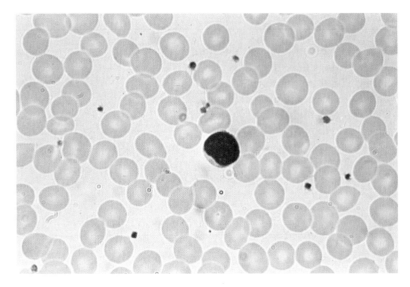

1.14. Mature lymphocytes
Blood film

Variable morphology in normal lymphocytes. All immunological types of lymphocyte circulate in the blood but do not have distinguishing features in their non-activated state.

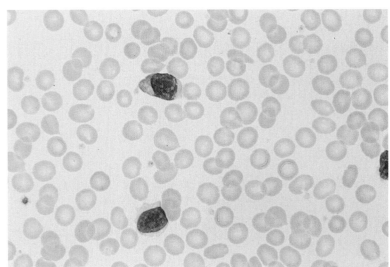

1.15. Plasma cell
Blood film

Plasma cells are only occasionally seen in children's blood. Activated forms may be present in response to infection.

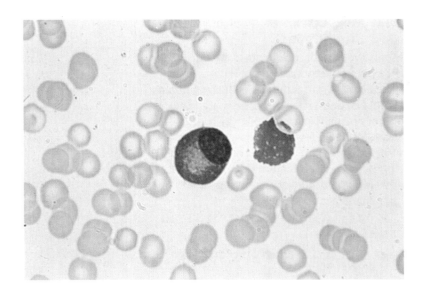

1.16. Megakaryocyte
Blood marrow

This is a mature megakaryocyte showing abundant granular cytoplasm and multiple nuclei. Platelets appear to be 'budding off' the cell.

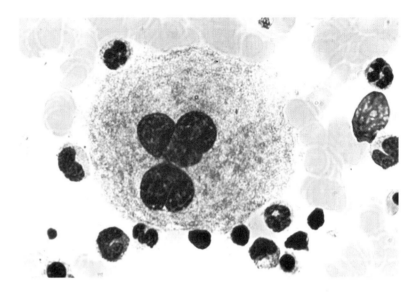

1.17. Normal iron stores
Bone marrow fragment; Perls' iron stain

Iron stores are stained blue and are contained within macrophages. (See red cell disorders—sideroblastic and megaloblastic sections).

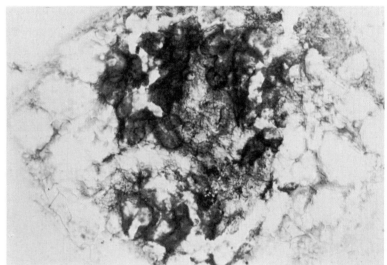

1.18. Osteoblasts
Bone marrow

These large mononuclear cells may be mistaken for tumour cells. They are more frequently encountered in children as marrow may easily be aspirated near an advancing zone of ossification.

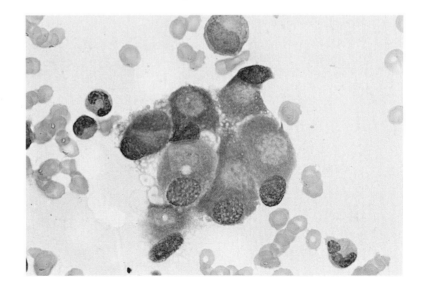

1.19. Osteoclast
Bone marrow

A large multinucleate cell which can be
mistaken for an atypical megakaryocyte or
a malignant syncytium.

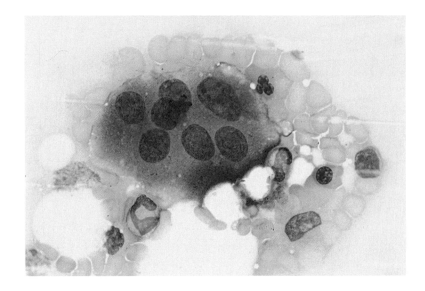

1.20. Normal marrow histology
Trephine biopsy

Overall cellularity varies, but tends to be
greater in children. In infancy, fat spaces
may be reduced to the point when
normality may be mistaken for a
myeloproliferative state. This section is
from a healthy four-month-old infant.

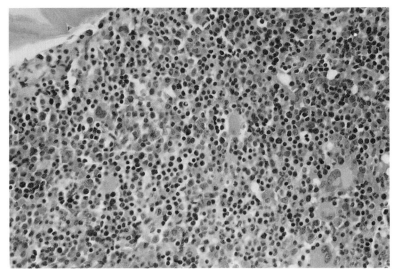

1.21. Normal marrow histology
Trephine biopsy

As 1.20 but from a normal four-year-old
child, to show variable cellularity.

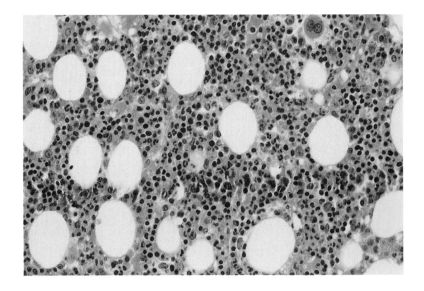

2
Congenital red cell disorders

2.1. Hereditary spherocytosis
Blood film

Blood film from a six-year-old boy presenting with jaundice and anaemia. His mother had a similar history.

Numerous microspherocytes are present. The larger reticulocytes are also seen.

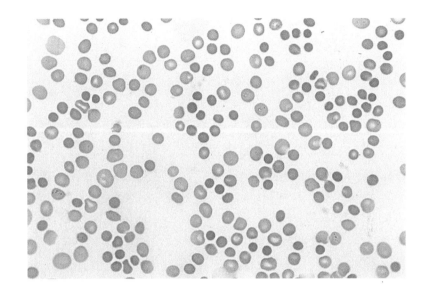

2.2. Hereditary haemolytic elliptocytosis
Blood film

This shows marked poikilocytosis with bizarre red cell shapes, fragmentation, micro-ovalocytes, and occasional spherocytes. An occasional typical elliptocyte may be seen. Between 10 and 15 per cent of patients with elliptocytosis present with clinical and laboratory evidence of haemolysis.

This patient was aged 18 months and had presented with neonatal jaundice. An erroneous diagnosis of 'infantile pyknocytosis' was made. His father had a similar blood picture.

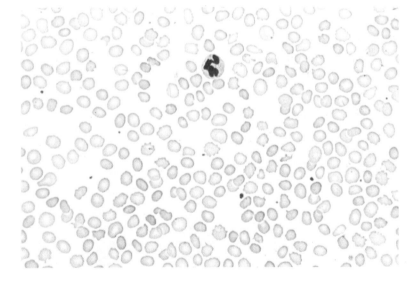

2.3. Hereditary elliptocytosis
Blood film

A majority of the red cells are elliptical in shape but there is no polychromasia. The patient inherited this autosomal dominant condition from his father but neither had evidence of haemolysis.

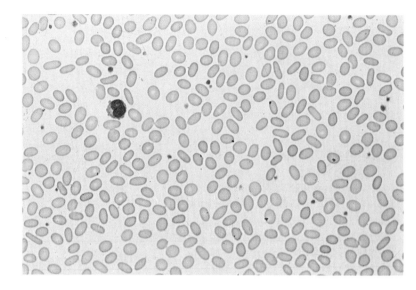

2.4. Hereditary elliptocytosis
Blood; high power

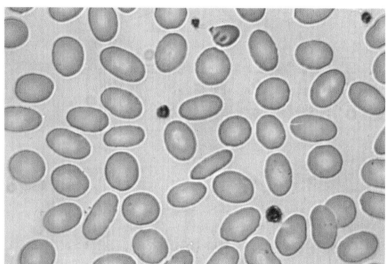

2.5. Hereditary stomatocytosis
Blood film

These red cells, with a central slit-like pale area, are typical of this condition. The same red cell appearances can be acquired in patients on intravenous feeding, with liver disease, or with a red cell sodium pump defect.

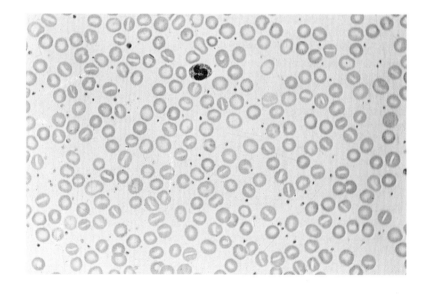

2.6. Hereditary stomatocytosis
Blood; high power

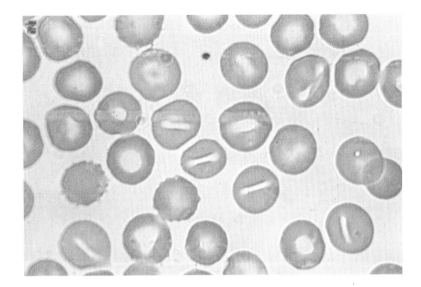

2.7. A-β-lipoproteinaemia
Blood film

This plate shows many 'spur cells' (acanthocytes). These cells can also be seen in liver disease, after splenectomy, and with certain malabsorption syndromes. Coarser 'burr cells' are seen in acute renal failure.

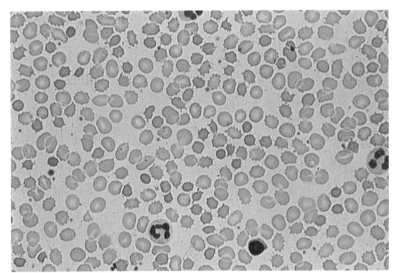

2.8. Hereditary pyropoikilocytosis
Blood film

The illustration shows extreme poikilocytosis with fragments, spherocytes, elliptocytes, 'triangulocytes', and other bizarre red cell forms. Macrocytes (reticulocytes) indicate the continuing severe chronic haemolytic process characteristic of this very rare disorder. The red cells are, as the name implies, sensitive to heat, their membranes 'fragmenting' at 45–46°C. Transfusion dependency is common but there is frequently a favourable response to splenectomy. The differential diagnosis of this blood film is from disseminated intravascular coagulation (in which the platelets would be low) and homozygous hereditary elliptocytosis. Recently a spectrin abnormality has been demonstrated.

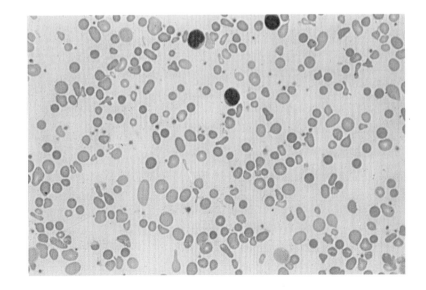

2.9. Pyruvate kinase deficiency
Blood film

Blood film from a two-year-old presenting with a Hb of 5.0 g/dl and reticulocytes of 30 per cent. In this disorder there is usually only slight anisopoikilocytosis but sometimes an irregularly contracted cell may be seen. This plate shows a 'spicule' or 'Sputnik' cell. In addition, acanthocytes may be seen.

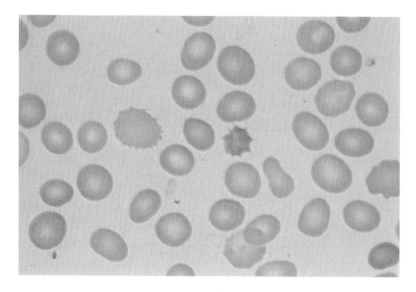

2.10. Favism
Blood film

Several red cells show 'puddling' of their haemoglobin with a residual thin rim of cytoplasm. Some red cell fragmentation and polychromasia are also seen.

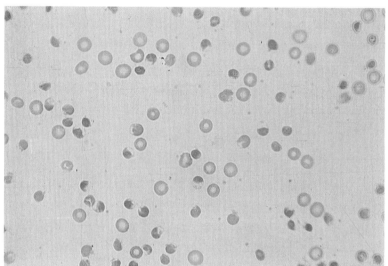

2.11. Favism
Blood; high power (see 2.10)

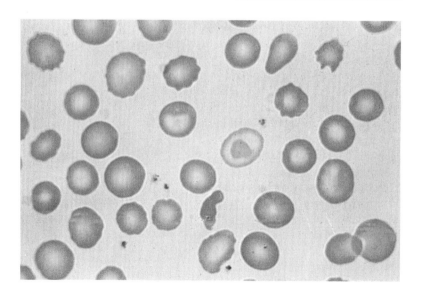

2.12. Pyrimidine-5′-nucleotidase deficiency
Blood film
This shows characteristically prominent basophilic stippling with marked polychromasia. This is a rare autosomal recessive disorder. The patient had a mild haemolytic anaemia with the haemoglobin varying in the range 8–10 g/dl.

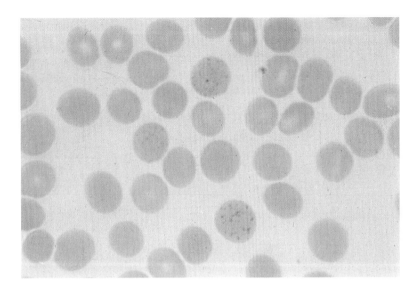

2.13. Hb Bart's Hydrops syndrome (Homozygous α′-thalassaemia)
Blood film
Cord blood from a hydropic and stillborn 32-week Singalese infant whose parents both had α′-thalassaemia trait. There are many normoblasts and marked anisocytosis. Hypochromia is only moderate but nearly all the haemoglobin is physiologically non-functional Hb Bart's (70–80 per cent) and Hb H with only traces of embryonic haemoglobins. Hbs A and F are absent. The nucleated red cells are bizarre and binucleate forms are frequent.

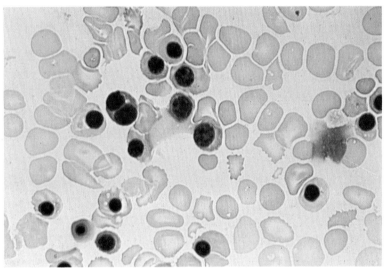

2.14. Hb Bart's Hydrops syndrome
Blood (see 2.13)

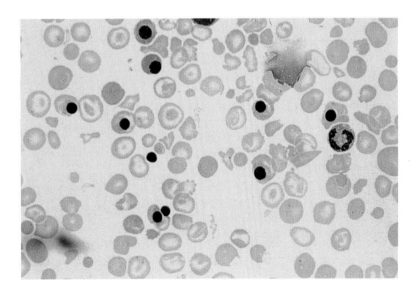

2.15. Hb H disease (α-thalassaemia)
Blood film

This 14-year-old boy has a compensated haemolytic anaemia and moderate splenomegaly. There is marked anisocytosis with many poikilocytes and some target cells. The reticulocyte count is 10–20 per cent. The red cells are hypochromic and microcytic because Hb production is reduced. Hb electrophoresis shows 70–80 per cent Hb A with 10–20 per cent fast-migrating Hb H, normal levels of Hb A_2, and a trace of Hb Bart's. Hb H is unstable (see 2.16).

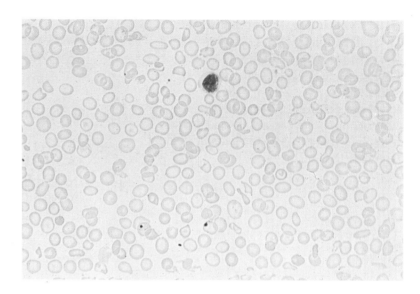

2.16. Hb H preparation
Blood film

In vitro incubation with methyl violet causes precipitation of Hb H as multiple dark-staining spots—a 'golf ball' appearance. (Same patient as 2.15.)

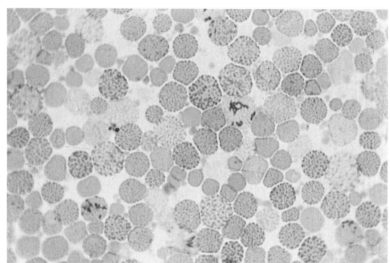

2.17. β-thalassaemia major
Blood film

Blood film from a newly-presenting Greek patient. There is marked hypochromia and red cell fragmentation though some normochromic red cells are seen. Nucleated red cells are present. Haemoglobin electrophoresis shows a normal or high-normal Hb A_2 level and up to 95 per cent Hb F. Hb A may be absent (β°-thalassaemia) or present at concentrations in the 2–20 per cent range (β⁺-thalassaemia). Kleihauer stain shows uneven distribution of Hb F between red cells.

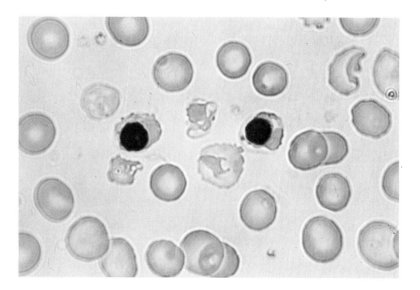

2.18. β-thalassaemia major (untreated)
Blood film

This patient also has folate deficiency. A giant metamyelocyte (see Section 3) is present. Beside it is a dysplastic normoblast showing marked hypochromia. Folate deficiency is secondary to the high red cell turnover resulting from breakdown of inclusion-damaged cells.

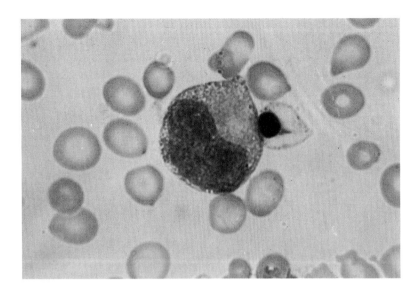

2.19. β-thalassaemia major post-splenectomy
Blood film

More hypochromic red cells are seen. Some contain Howell—Jolly bodies. There is also a giant platelet (see Section 3; post-splenectomy). Methyl violet stain would show many more α-chain inclusions which, prior to splenectomy, would have been 'culled-out' by the spleen.

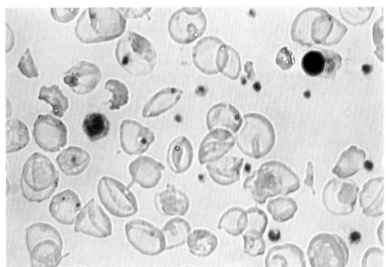

2.20. Thalassaemia intermedia
Blood film

There is marked anisocytosis and hypochromia. No nucleated red cells are seen. Clinically intermediate thalassaemia has many causes including δ-β-thalassaemia homozygosity and interaction of β-thalassaemia with HPFH and α-thalassaemia. Such patients are, by definition, not transfusion dependent but do have chronic haemolysis.

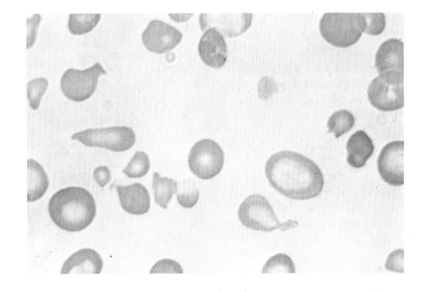

2.21. β-thalassaemia minor (or trait)
Blood film

There is anisocytosis and red cells are microcytic and hypochromic. Target cells and occasional fragmented cells are seen. The major differential diagnosis is iron deficiency. Hb electrophoresis shows increased Hb A_2 (unless there is coexistent iron deficiency) and, in 60–70 per cent of cases, a slightly raised Hb F.

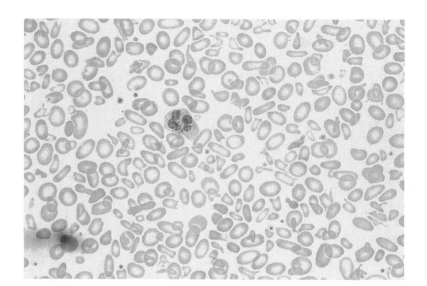

2.22. Homozygous δ-β-thalassaemia
Blood film; Kleihauer stain

This 10-year-old boy had thalassaemia intermedia and Hb electrophoresis showed 100 per cent Hb F. Homozygosity for the HPFH gene was excluded by (a) the child's Arab origin; (b) parental studies; and (c) a demonstration of a marked reduction of γ-compared with α-chain synthesis by his reticulocytes. The apparent heterogeneity of Hb F between red cells is a result of each cell's varying Hb content.

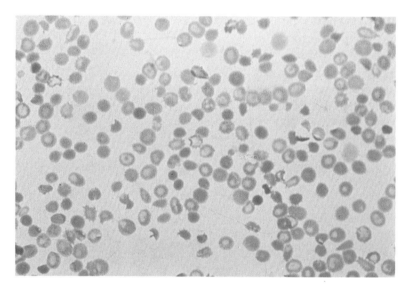

2.23. β-thalassaemia major
Bone marrow

These plates show erythroid hyperplasia and iron-laden macrophages. In 2.23 there are brown siderotic granules, which in 2.24 are confirmed as iron by Perls' stain.

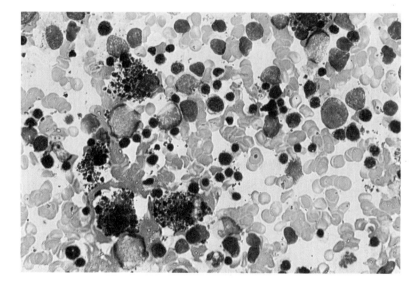

2.24. β-thalassaemia major
Bone marrow; Perls' stain (see 2.23)

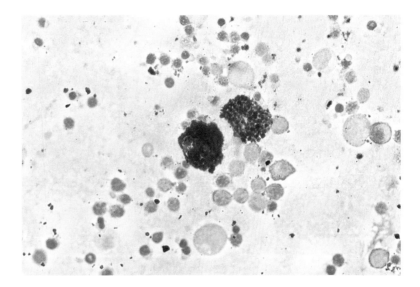

2.25. Sickle-cell anaemia
Blood film

This child—a West Indian aged 10 years—presented with hip pain and pneumonia. He was in a sickle-cell crisis. Numerous sickled cells are present. Hb electrophoresis showed predominant Hb S with 5 per cent Hb F and a normal Hb A$_2$ level and no Hb A.

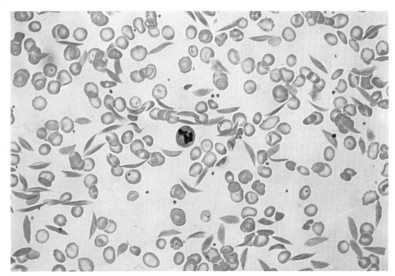

2.26. Sickle β-thalassaemia
Blood film

One sickled cell and many target cells are seen. The red cells are hypochromic. Hb electrophoresis shows 0–20 per cent Hb A; 30–40 per cent Hb F; 40–50 per cent Hb S; and normal or increased Hb A$_2$.

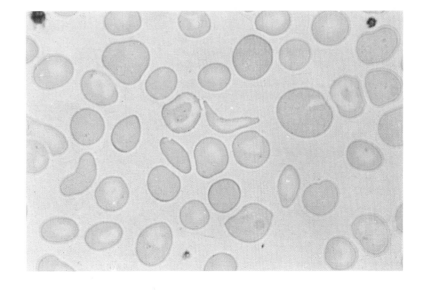

2.27. Hb S-C disease
Blood film

This West African patient, aged six years, was admitted because of a painful sickling crisis. Electrophoresis of patient and parental Hb confirmed the diagnosis. The blood film, showing sickled cells and prominent target cells, together with polychromasia, is characteristic.

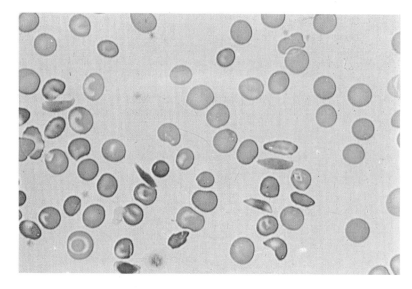

2.28. Hb S-C disease
Blood film (cont. from 2.27)

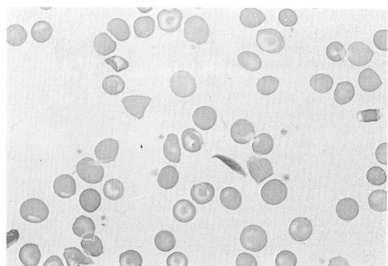

2.29. Hb C trait
Blood film

Many of the red cells are target forms. In homozygous Hb C disease all the red cells are target cells. (See also Hb E trait; 2.30.)

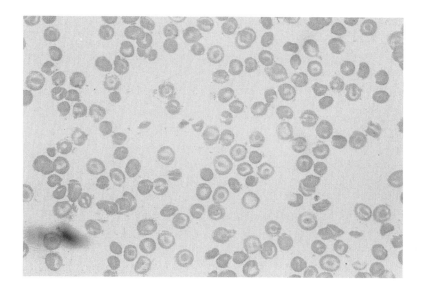

2.30. Hb E trait
Blood film

Blood film from an Indian child. The red cells are normochromic and target cells are present; differentiation from Hb C trait is by the patient's ethnic origin and by Hb electrophoresis.

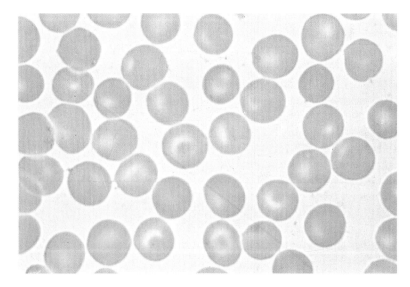

2.31 and 2.32. Hb E-thalassaemia
Blood film

There is marked anisocytosis and hypochromia. A dysplastic nucleated red cell is seen in 2.32 and target cells are frequent. These patients are almost always transfusion dependent.

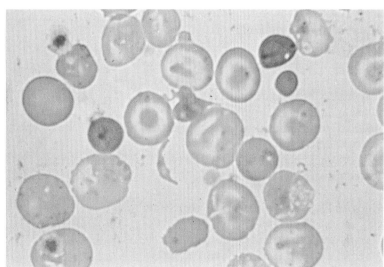

2.32. Hb E-thalassemia
Blood film. See 2.31

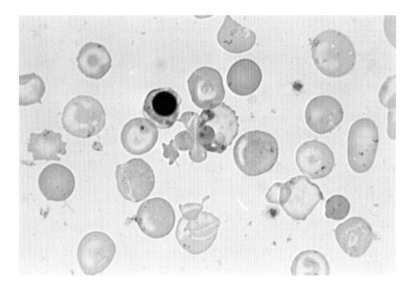

2.33. Unstable haemoglobin (Hb Hammersmith)
Blood film

The MGG film shows a marked anisocytosis with polychromasia. There are poikilocytes and the red cell in the centre of the field has prominent basophilic stippling. There are about 50 unstable variants of Hb. Under stress these Hb's denature easily, precipitate within the cells and form Heinz bodies. These rigid inclusions cause premature red cell destruction in the spleen. The consequent haemolytic anaemia may be severe (Hb Hammersmith or Hb Bristol) or mild to moderate (Hb Köln).

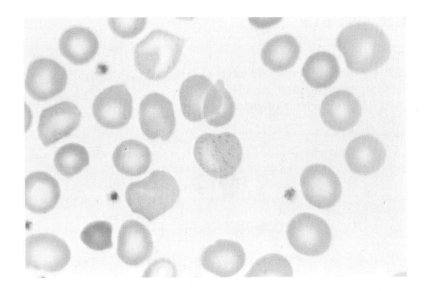

2.34. Haemolytic anaemia due to unstable Hb Köln
Blood film

This is an unstable haemoglobin resulting in a congenital Heinz-body haemolytic anaemia (cf. 2.35). Affected patients have a congenital non-spherocytic haemolytic anaemia, which in this case is of moderate severity. Splenectomy may be of value and oxidant drugs must be avoided. The blood film shows the presence of basophilic inclusions (arrowed), which in this instance were usually single, although in other cases they are multiple. The red cells are hypochromic with some crenation but spherocytes are usually only present during a haemolytic crisis.

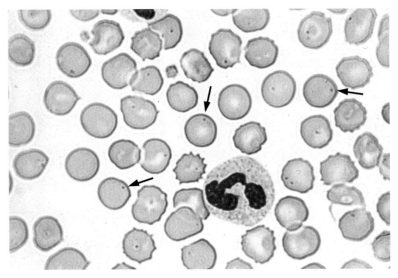

2.35 (a). Unstable haemoglobin
Blood film; Heinz body preparation

This supravital stain using methyl violet shows Heinz bodies as dark, round precipitates in the red cells. The bodies are attached to the cell membrane. The blood is from the same patient as in 2.33. Heinz bodies are more plentiful after splenectomy.

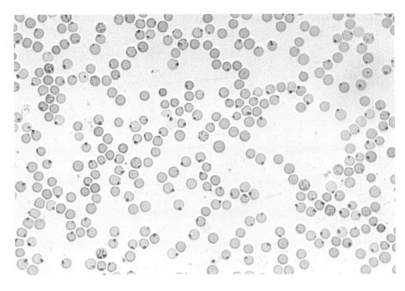

2.35 (b). Unstable haemoglobin

Blood film; Heinz body
preparation

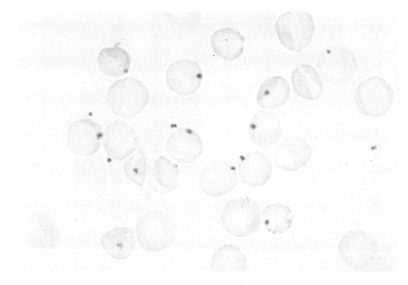

2.36. Congenital erythropoietic porphyria

Bone marrow (UV fluorescence)
The normoblasts in this condition contain
uroporphyrin I which fluoresces intensely
under UV light at 400 nm. The disease
presents in early childhood with destructive
skin lesions in areas exposed to sunlight
and with hirsutism and hyperpigmentation.
The patient's urine is red or pink. These
features have been suggested as the origin
for the 'werewolf' stories.

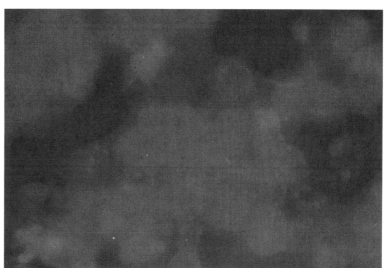

2.37, 2.38, and 2.39. Diamond–Blackfan syndrome

Bone marrow
Red cell precursors are virtually absent.
Iron-laden macrophages are seen (2.38)
and the iron stain (2.39) shows increased
stores.

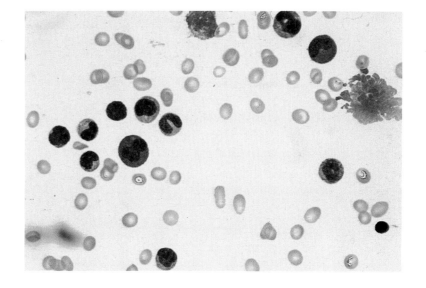

2.38. Diamond–Blackfan syndrome
Bone marrow (see 2.37)
Iron laden macrophages are present.

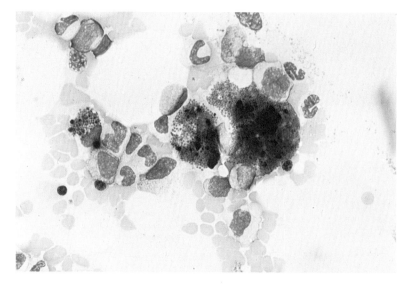

2.39. Diamond–Blackfan syndrome
Bone marrow (Perls' iron stain)

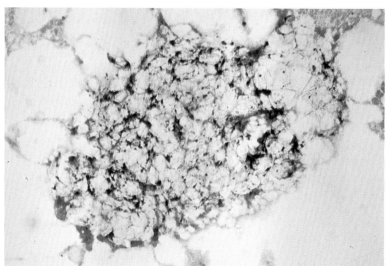

2.40 and 2.41. Congenital dyserythropoietic anaemia (CDA) type I
Blood film
There is marked anisocytosis with polychromasia. 'Helmet cells', 'tadpole cells', and small fragments are seen.

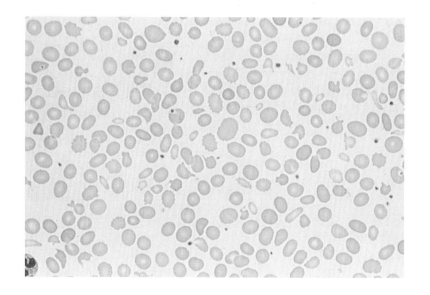

2.41. CDA type I
Blood film. See 2.40

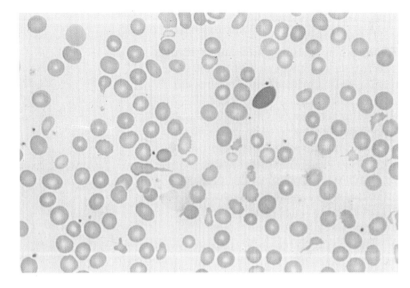

2.42. CDA type I
Blood film
Examples of red cell fragmentation.

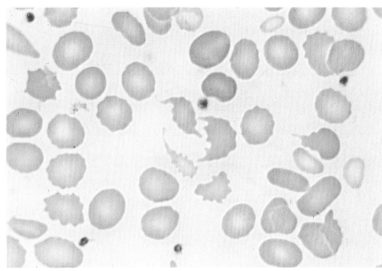

2.43. CDA type I
Blood film
Intense basophilic stippling in a red cell.

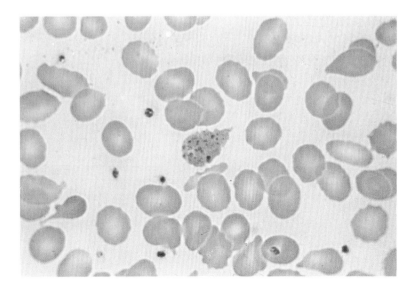

2.44, 2.45, 2.46, and 2.47. CDA type I
  Bone marrow

All the plates show characteristic erythroid hyperplasia with megaloblastosis and giant metamyelocytes. Diagnostic features are internuclear bridging—a strand of chromatin between two nuclei (2.44, 2.45); basophilic stippling in normoblasts (2.46); and abnormal nuclear pyknosis in normoblasts (2.47). No serological abnormalities are present. The patient presented with anaemia, splenomegaly, and a slightly raised bilirubin. Diagnosis may be delayed until adolescence.

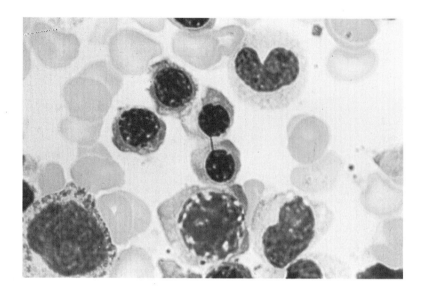

2.45. CDA type I
  Bone marrow
Internuclear bridging.

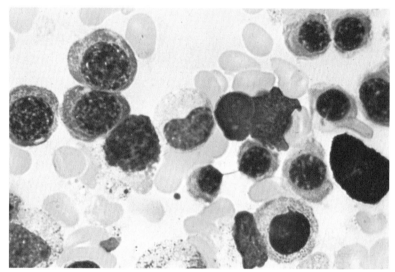

2.46. CDA type I
  Bone marrow
Basophilic stippling in two normoblasts.

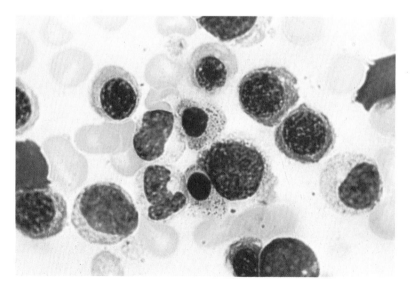

2.47. CDA type I
Bone marrow
A normoblast pyknotic nucleus.

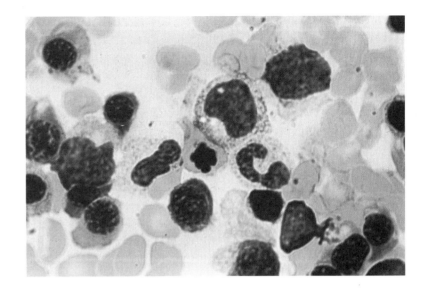

2.48. CDA type II, 'HEMPAS'
Blood film
This shows less anisocytosis and poikilocytosis than the CDA I blood film.

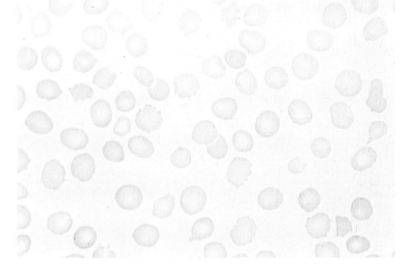

2.49. CDA type II
Bone marrow
This low-power view shows erythroid hyperplasia. Multinuclearity is prominent and present in the late erythroblasts. There are few internuclear bridges. Megaloblastic changes are not as marked as in CDA type I. This is the commonest CDA and is diagnosed by a positive acid serum lysis (Ham's test) as well as by the morphological changes. The patient, aged eight years, presented with a mild anaemia, mild jaundice, and hepatosplenomegaly. She also had gallstones.

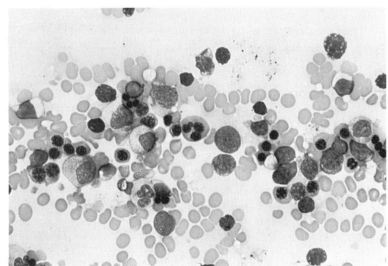

2.50, 2.51, 2.52, and 2.53. CDA type II
Bone marrow
High-power views showing in more detail the bizarre appearances of red cell precursors.

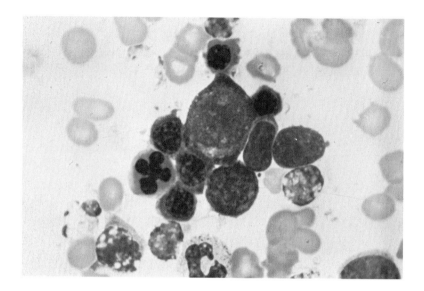

2.51. CDA type II
Bone marrow
Multinucleate red cell precursors.

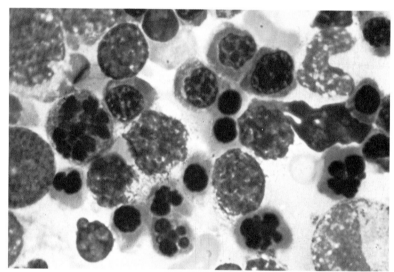

2.52. CDA type II
Bone marrow
Iron-laden macrophage.

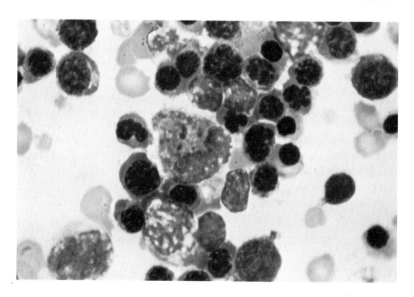

2.53. CDA type II
Bone marrow (see 2.50)

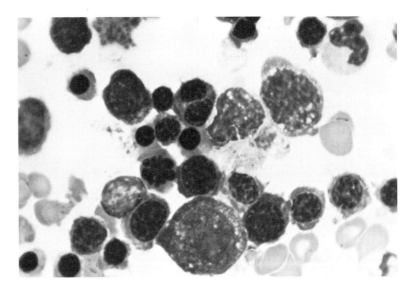

2.54. CDA type III
Blood film

There is marked poikilocytosis, macrocytosis, and polychromasia. This is the rarest form of CDA. Diagnosis may be delayed until adult life and patients present with anaemia. The liver and spleen may be palpable.

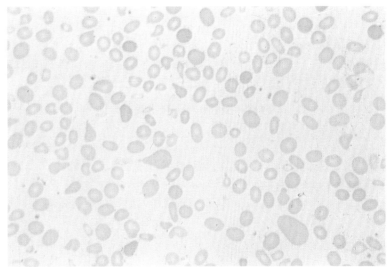

2.55. CDA type III
Blood film

Marked red cell basophilic stippling.

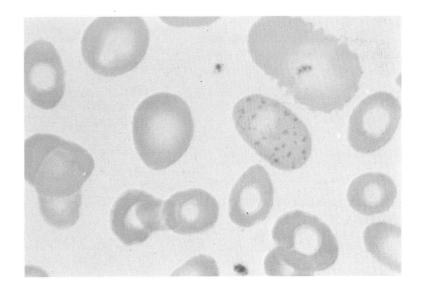

2.56. CDA type III
Bone marrow

This low-power view shows intense erythroid activity with many multinucleate cells. The next three plates show in more detail the multinuclearity, basophilic stippling, and nuclear lobulation. Multinuclearity is sometimes so striking that the cells are called 'gigantoblasts'.

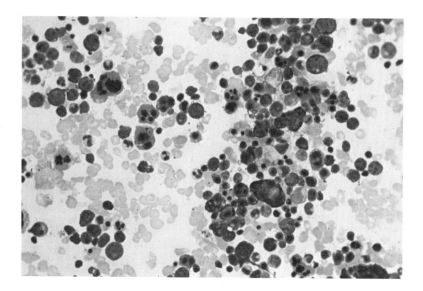

2.57. CDA type III
Bone marrow; high power

Nuclear lobulation and multinucleate cells.

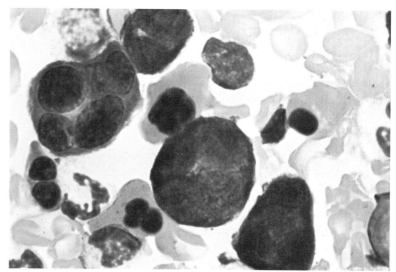

2.58. CDA type III
Bone marrow; high power

Multinuclearity and basophilic stippling.

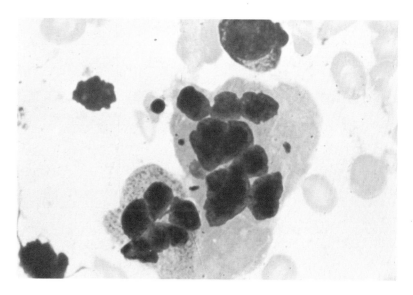

2.59. CDA type III
Bone marrow; high power
'Gigantoblasts' (see 2.56).

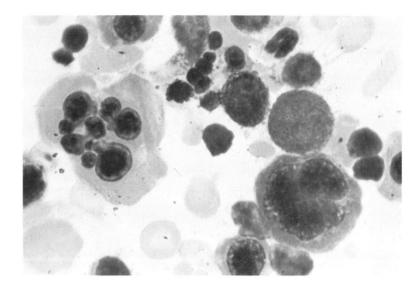

2.60 and 2.61. Hereditary sideroblastic anaemia (post-transfusion)
Blood film

This shows many hypochromic microcytes.
The normochromic cells may be residual
transfused cells. In 2.61 the marrow shows
ring sideroblasts. This is inherited as a sex-
linked recessive disorder. The bone
marrow is normoblastic.

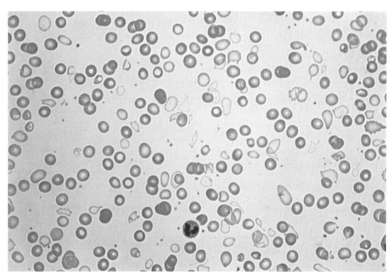

2.61. Hereditary sideroblastic anaemia
Marrow; iron stain

Ring sideroblasts are present in
normoblastic marrow.

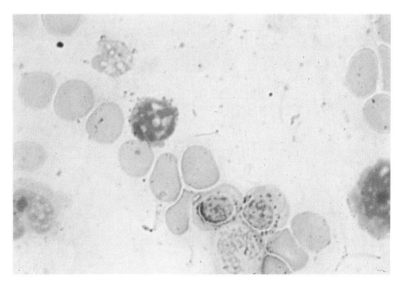

2.62 and 2.63. Fanconi's anaemia— dyserythropoiesis
Bone marrow

Both plates show abnormal red cell precursors—here a 'trefoil' nucleated red cell. The patient was a two-year-old girl who also had a congenital heart defect and abnormal forearms. She had a normal Hb and white cell count but was thrombocytopenic. She later developed complete marrow aplasia.

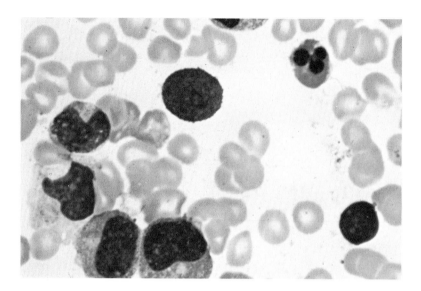

2.63. Fanconi's anaemia
Bone marrow

Abnormal vacuolation of red cell precursors (arrow); this is also said to occur in some cases of chloramphenicol myelotoxicity and Schwachman–Diamond syndrome.

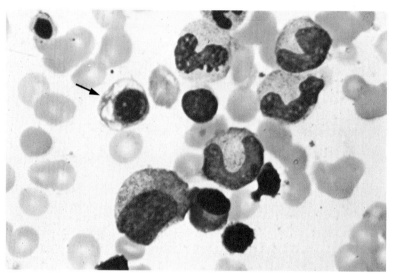

3
Acquired and secondary red cell disorders

3.1. Simple iron lack
Blood film

Haemoglobin 6.6 g/dl; MCV 55 fl, MCH 12 pg; gross hypochromia and microcytosis. Haemoglobin A_2 concentration normal. Five-year-old Asian child with gross dietary deficiency, a particular problem for this ethnic group.

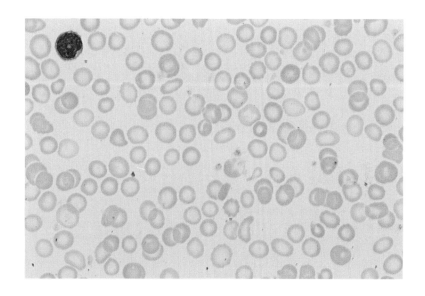

3.2. Iron lack with co-existent β-thalassaemia trait
Blood film

Haemoglobin 8.8 g/dl; ferritin 3 μg/l; haemoglobin A_2 5.5 per cent, F 2.6 per cent. Asian child with dietary deficiency. Thalassaemia trait in this ethnic group not infrequently associates with iron deficiency and the two are not mutually exclusive.

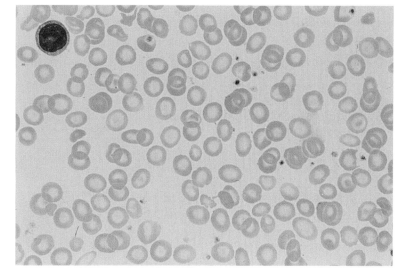

3.3. Iron lack due to bleeding
Blood film

Haemoglobin 6.1 g/dl. Asian child returned from Pakistan with heavy infestation of hookworm (*Ankylostoma duodenale*). The patient also had a marked eosinophilia—1.2 × 10⁹/l.

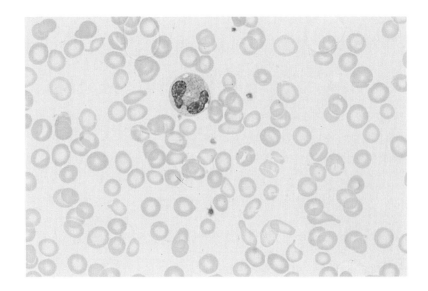

3.4. Partially treated iron lack
Blood film

Six days iron supplements to a starting haemoglobin of 5.4 g/dl; rise of concentration to 6.7 g/dl. Dimorphic picture; note larger polychromatic cells emerging.

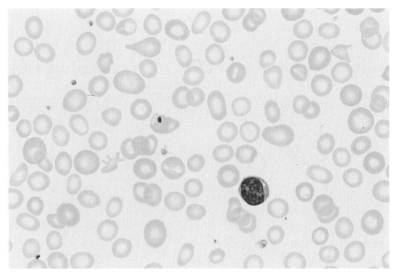

3.5. Megaloblastic anaemia—dietary folate deficiency
Blood film

Gross anisocytosis with normochromic oval macrocytes. MCV 102 fl; serum folate 0.2 μg/l; red cell folate 65 μg/l (lower limit of normal 2 and 170 μg respectively). Four-year-old girl, anorexic following cancer chemotherapy.

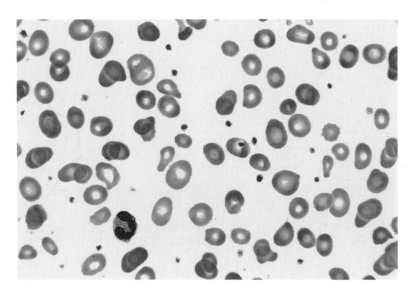

3.6. Megaloblastic anaemia—dietary folate deficiency
Blood film

Child of 10 months with strict vegan parents and diet deficient in vitamin B_{12} and folate. Hypersegmented neutrophils of this type are seen in all varieties of macrocytic anaemia that result from megaloblastic haemopoiesis.

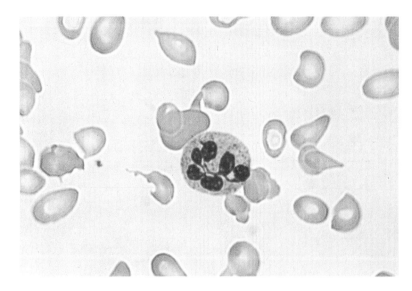

3.7. Megaloblastic anaemia— marrow appearances (red cells)
Bone marrow

Intermediate and late megaloblasts, the latter showing orthochromasia, alongside polychromatic normoblasts. The marrow is from the child illustrated in 3.5.

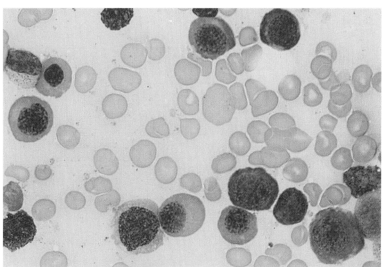

3.8. Megaloblastic anaemia— marrow appearances (white cells)
Bone marrow

Giant myelocytes and metamyelocytes. Note normal small lymphocyte as size marker. A two-year-old child with congenital deficiency of transcobalamin II.

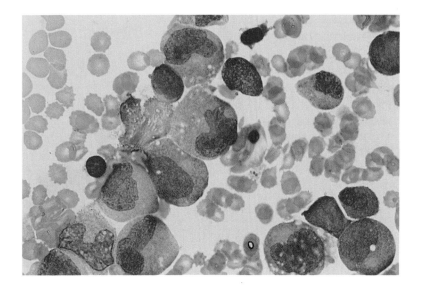

3.9. Megaloblastic anaemia—iron stores
Bone marrow; Perls' stain
Abundant stainable iron in marrow particle seen at low power.

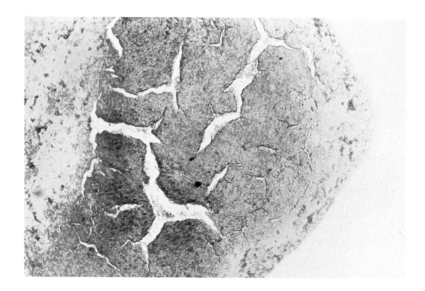

3.10. Megaloblastic anaemia— sideroblasts
Bone marrow; Perls' stain
Normal sideroblast staining is seen in most uncomplicated megaloblastic anaemias (arrowed cells). Ring sideroblasts are not a feature.

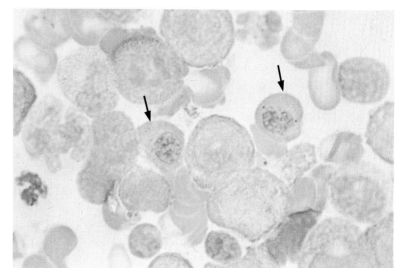

3.11. Megaloblastic anaemia— combined iron and folate deficiency
Bone marrow
Red cell megaloblastic changes are masked to some extent when iron deficiency co-exists, but giant metamyelocytes are still evident. From a child with gluten enteropathy.

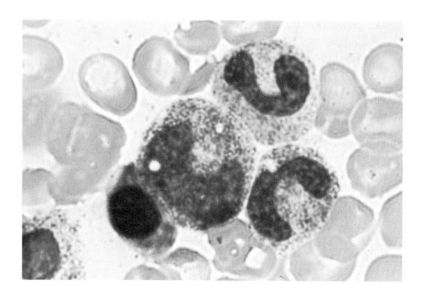

3.12. Coeliac disease
Blood film
In addition to features of folate deficiency (hypersegmented neutrophil), this example also shows evidence of associated hyposplenism—fragmented red cells and Howell–Jolly bodies.

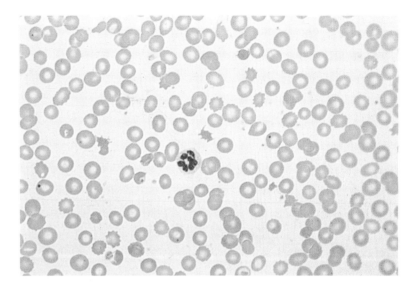

3.13. Lead poisoning
Blood film
A red cell with prominent basophilic stippling is seen. Hypochromia was not particularly prominent in this instance. The two-year-old patient was investigated for anaemia and colic. He was seen to nibble at paint on a window frame.

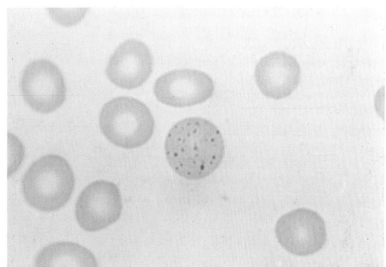

3.14. Chronic renal failure
Blood film
Haemoglobin 5.2 g/dl; normochromic and unremarkable red cells. Creatinine 1085 μmol/l; urea 49.2 mmol/l. MCV 83 fl; MCH 25.5, reticulocytopenia. Thirteen-year-old boy with obstructive uropathy at six months leading to nephrectomy on one side and a poorly functioning kidney on the other; undialysed.

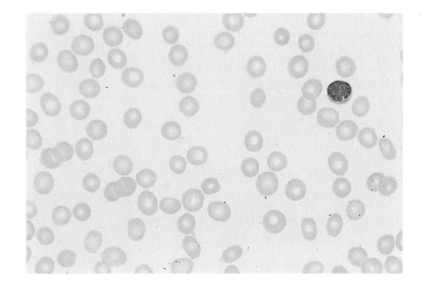

3.15. Chronic renal failure
Blood film

Seven-year-old child with congenital dysplastic kidneys on long-term peritoneal dialysis. Haemoglobin 8.8 g/dl; MCV 90 fl; MCH 30.9 (untransfused). Minimal macrocytosis; red cells unremarkable.

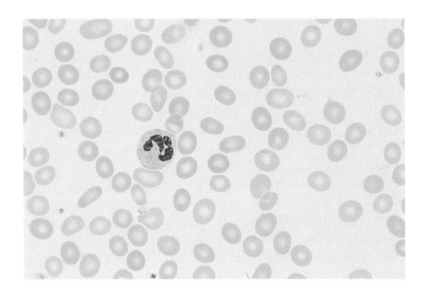

3.16. Liver disease—sepsis and intravascular coagulation
Blood film

Terminal hepatic failure in a child of 7 months with associated sepsis and intravascular coagulation. Bilirubin 52 μmol/l; ALT 423 u/l. Target cells, crenated cells, and irregularly contracted cells.

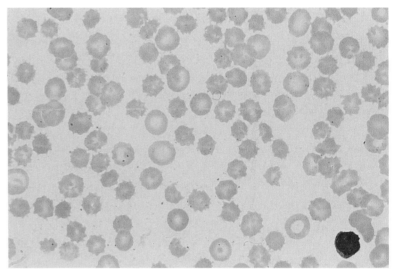

3.17. Liver disease—biliary atresia
Blood film

Biliary atresia in a five-year-old. Well, with progressive obstructive jaundice awaiting liver transplantation. Bilirubin 185 μmol/l; ALT 76 u/l; alkaline phosphatase 1206 u/l.

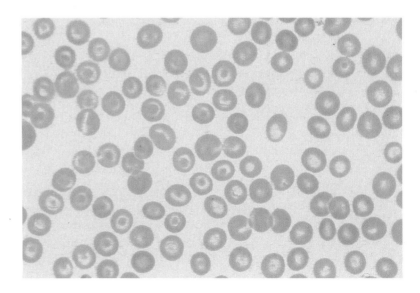

3.18. Liver disease—biliary atresia
Blood film
A further case of biliary atresia with more marked red cell changes—target cells, leptocytes.

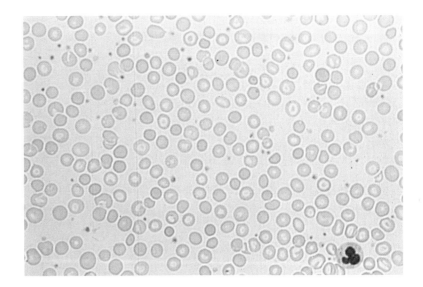

3.19. Transient erythroblastopenia of childhood
Blood film
Profound normochromic anaemia with absent or grossly reduced reticulocytes in an otherwise well child. Often there is an associated thrombocytosis. White cells are unremarkable.

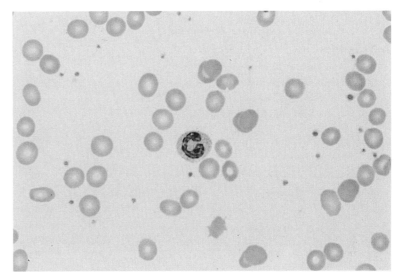

3.20. Transient erythroblastopenia of childhood
Bone marrow
Absent or grossly reduced erythroblasts. Granulopoiesis is unremarkable. The relative (or occasionally absolute) lymphocytosis can give rise to an erroneous diagnosis of lymphoblastic leukaemia.

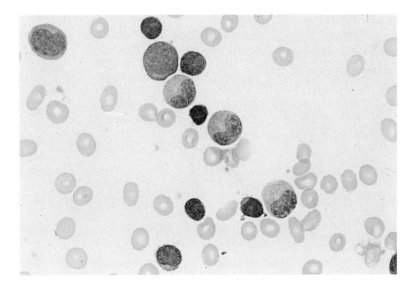

3.21. Acquired haemolytic anaemia—immune warm type
Blood film

Four-year-old with haemolysis complicating systemic lupus erythematosus. Haemoglobin 5 g/dl. Polychromasia and spherocytes.

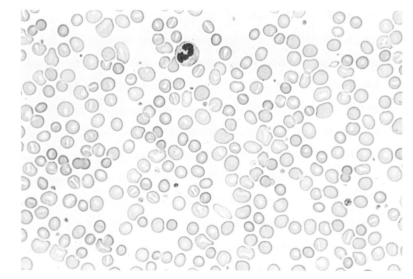

3.22. Acquired haemolytic anaemia—immune warm type
Blood film

Idiopathic autoimmune haemolysis with antibody showing anti-ē specificity. A five-year-old child with splenomegaly: haemoglobin 5.2 g/dl; MCV 94 fl; reticulocytes 610×10^9/l; and nucleated red cells 2.6×10^9/l. Gross anisocytosis, marked spherocytosis.

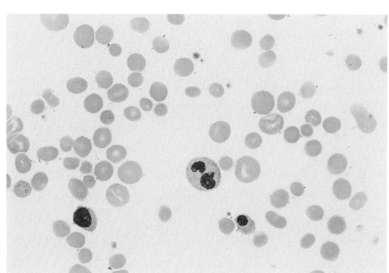

3.23. Acquired haemolytic anaemia—immune cold type
Blood film

Gross agglutination at room temperature in a seven-year-old boy with mycoplasma pneumonia. There was associated haemolysis with a haemoglobin of 8 g/dl, and a marked reticulocytosis. Direct AHG test was positive with the red cells being coated with C4, C3b and C3d. Serum contained a cold auto/panagglutinin with anti-I specificity.

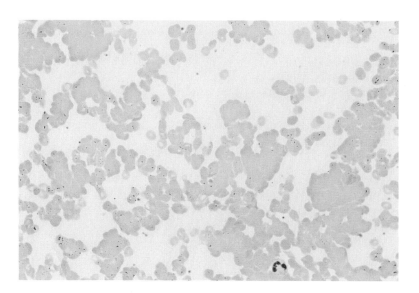

3.24. Acquired haemolytic anaemia—paroxysmal cold haemoglobinuria
Blood film

PCH is occasionally seen in children following virus infections as an episode of acute haemolysis associated with the Donath–Landsteiner antibody with anti-P specificity. There are microagglutinates and there is erythrophagocytosis by neutrophils.

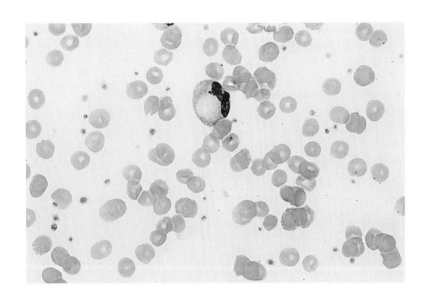

3.25. Secondary haemolytic anaemia—haemolytic uraemic syndrome
Blood film

Marked red cell fragmentation associated with anaemia, thrombocytopenia, and renal failure but in the absence of disseminated intravascular coagulation. Girl of 5 years.

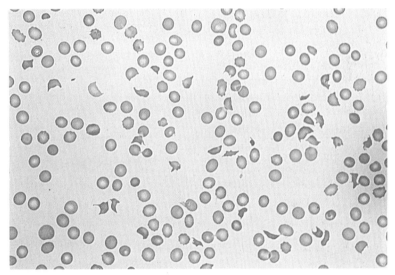

3.26. Secondary haemolytic anaemia—mechanical haemolysis
Blood film

Spherocytes, fragmented cells and polychromasia. Platelet count and renal function normal. A nine-year-old with a Teflon graft to repair a ventricular septal defect.

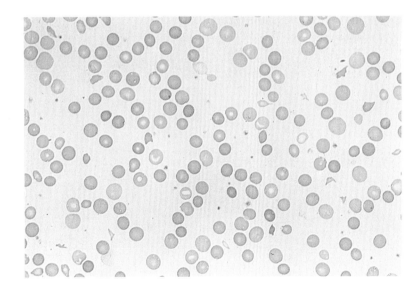

3.27. Secondary haemolytic anaemia—giant haemangioma
Blood film
The Kasabach–Merritt syndrome, producing a microangiopathic haemolytic state due to the pathological microcirculation in the lesion. Red cell fragmentation and spherocytes are associated with thrombocytopenia.

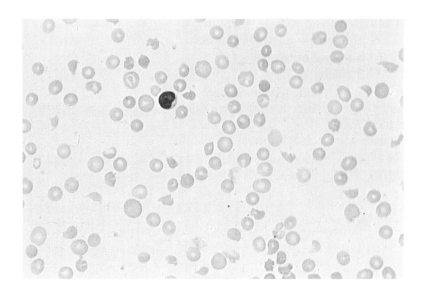

3.28. Secondary haemolytic anaemia—extensive burns
Blood film
The film has a 'dirty' appearance due to cell debris and proteinaceous material. Partially burnt red cells have sphered, and others have completely lysed. Haemoglobin 6.2 g/dl. Six-month-old child in house fire.

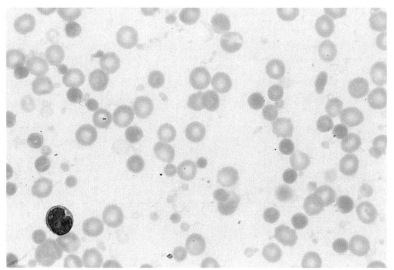

3.29. Haemolytic anaemia—reticulocyte stain
Reticulocyte preparation
Taken from the patient illustrated in 3.21.

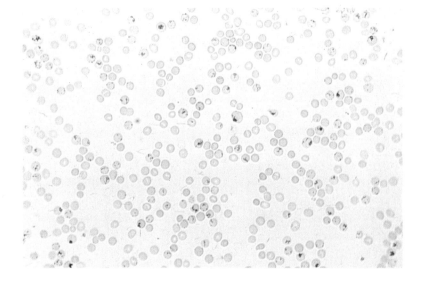

3.30. Haemolytic anaemia—bone marrow
Bone marrow
Normoblastic hyperplasia is the normal response to haemolysis from any cause. Its absence does not preclude haemolysis, nor does its presence necessarily indicate it.

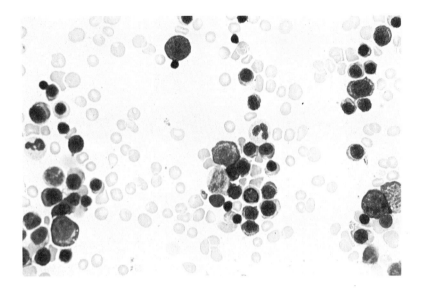

3.31. Post-splenectomy changes
Blood film
Anisocytosis, poikilocytosis, target cells, thrombocytosis and Howell–Jolly bodies. Twelve-year-old splenectomized for immune neutropenia.

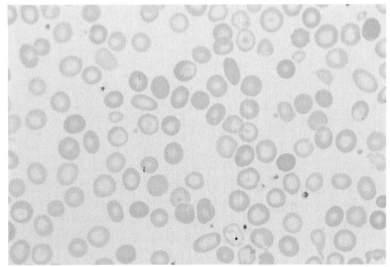

3.32. Congenital absence of spleen
Blood film
Burr cells, target cells, Howell–Jolly bodies and polychromasia. A 10-month-old boy with an associated congenital heart defect—hypoplastic right outflow tract and partial situs inversus.

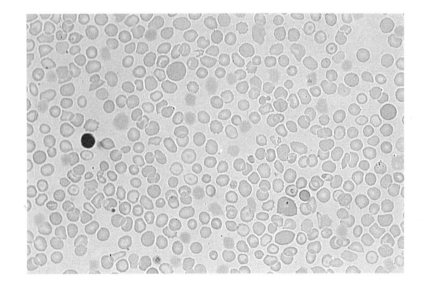

4
Disorders of polymorphonuclear leucocytes

4.1. Toxic granulation of neutrophils
Blood film

Dense neutrophil cytoplasmic granules are present and probably represent increased lysosomal content. There is a 'left shift' with reduced lobulation of the neutrophil nuclei. These features are present in patients with infections and other stresses (compare Section 14).

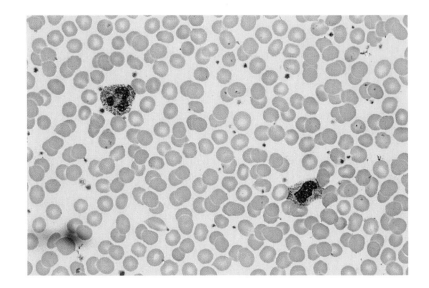

4.2. Toxic change due to septicaemia
Bone marrow

Toxic granulation is present in all the polymorph precursors and there is an increase in more primitive forms such as myelocytes and promyelocytes giving a so-called 'left shift'.

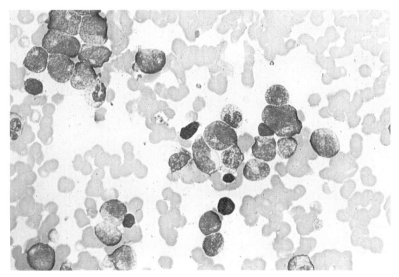

4.3. Pelger—Hüet anomaly
Blood film
This anomaly is transmitted in autosomal dominant fashion. Nuclei may be bilobed or oval-shaped.

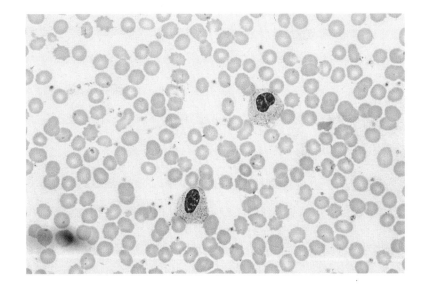

4.4. Pelger—Hüet anomaly
High-power blood film
The 'pince-nez' appearance of the neutrophils is shown in this plate. Neutrophils resembling these may also be seen in several acquired diseases such as myeloproliferative disorders and during sulphonamide therapy.

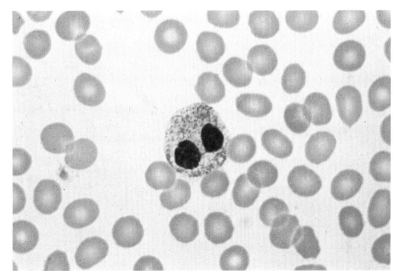

4.5. Neutrophil alkaline phosphatase (NAP)
Blood film; stain see ref. 6
NAP activity is located in secondary and tertiary neutrophil granules and can be demonstrated by an azo-dye coupling technique. The intensity of brown stain is an approximate measure of the cells' content of enzyme. The normal range in older patients is 35–100, scoring intensity of individual cells from 0–4 and counting 100 consecutive neutrophils. However, the scores tend to be higher in children with a neonatal range of 150–300. High scores also occur in infections, Down's syndrome, and leukaemoid reactions. Low scores are found in CGL in relapse, myeloblastic leukaemias, aplastic anaemia, and infectious mononucleosis.

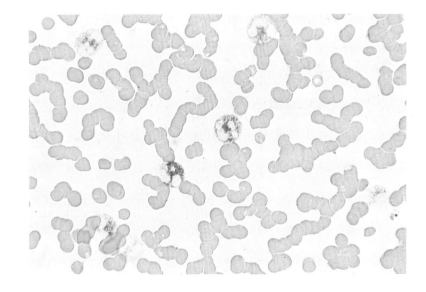

4.6. LE preparation
Blood film; stain see ref. 18
Neutrophils have ingested nuclear material which displaces the polymorph nucleus to the side of the cell. This process depends on an antinuclear IgG which is present in systemic lupus erythematosus and some other collagenoses. Its use has been superseded by DNA-binding and ANA-testing.

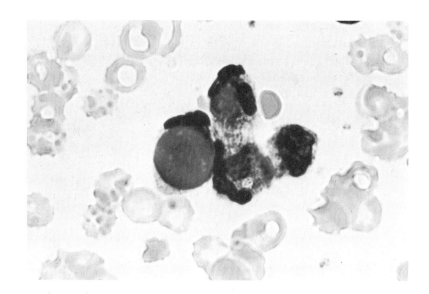

4.7. Eosinophilia due to toxoplasmosis
Blood film
Infection with *Toxoplasma gondii* is a cause of the 'infectious mononucleosis syndrome' in which generalized lymphadenopathy is associated with circulating atypical lymphocytes. In this case the more prominent feature was an eosinophilia. For a complete differential diagnosis of eosinophilia see ref. 20.

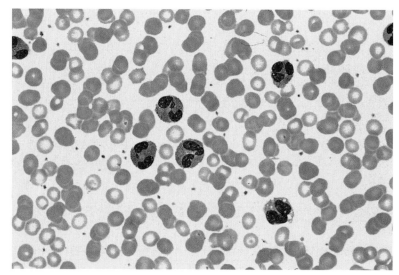

4.8. Chediak–Higashi syndrome
Blood film
Patients with this autosomal recessive trait present with oculocutaneous albinism, fine light hair, susceptibility to infection, and, sometimes, neurological problems and bleeding diathesis. The neutrophils (as shown here), other white cells, as well as other tissue cells show pyknotic nuclei and large irregular cytoplasmic granules.

This condition often progresses with pancytopenia and hepatosplenomegaly. Lymphoma-like disorders are also seen.

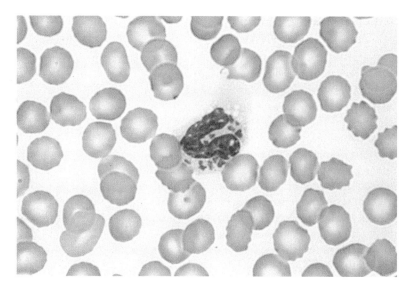

4.9. Chediak–Higashi syndrome
Electron micrograph
Neutrophil containing abnormal granulation corresponding to the irregular granules shown in 4.8.

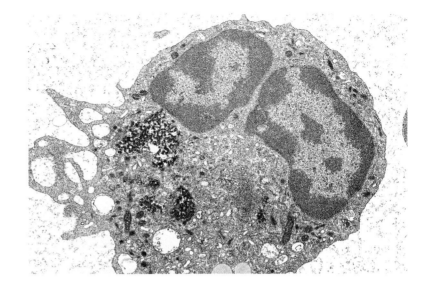

4.10. Chediak–Higashi syndrome
Bone marrow
The characteristic large eosinophilic granules are shown as well as the abnormal neutrophil granules.

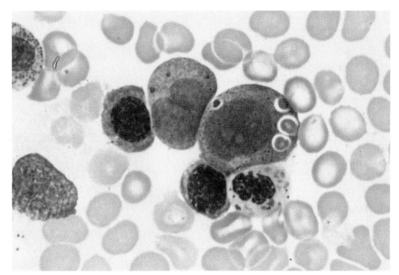

4.11. Nitro blue tetrazolium (NBT) test
Blood film; method see ref. 20
Neutrophils reduce the soluble redox dyes of tetrazolium salts to insoluble black formazan deposits. This reflects superoxide and singlet oxygen production by neutrophils during phagocytosis. The test can be used to detect both carriers and affected patients with chronic granulomatous disease.

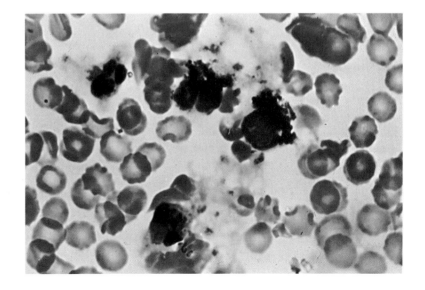

4.12. Opsonization experiment; positive result
Blood film

Normal serum provokes complete ingestion of yeast granules by phagocytes. This function is dependent upon two types of serum factor, IgG and C3, which coat the particles or bacteria.

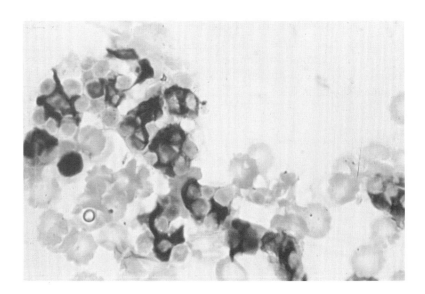

4.13. Opsonization experiment; negative result
Blood film

Failure of yeast phagocytosis in this set of experimental conditions occurs when there is a deficiency of C2, C3 or C5, or a specific defect of humoral immunity. Recurrent and chronic pyogenic infections commonly result.

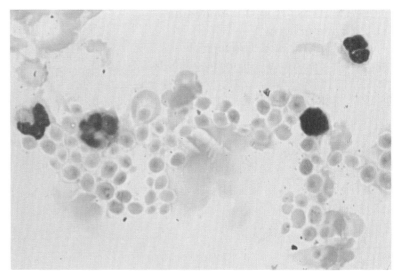

4.14. Systemic mastocytosis
Bone marrow

The sample is from a three-year-old girl with moderate hepatosplenomegaly and developmental delay. She presented at age 13 months with fits sometimes associated with fever. She is said to have been 'flushed' at birth, perhaps as a result of histamine release from mast cells during the birth process.

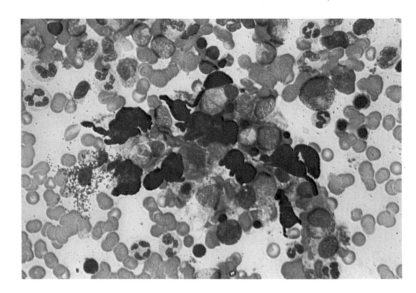

4.15. Systemic mastocytosis
  Bone marrow; toluidine blue;
  ref. 12(a)
Same patient as in 4.14.

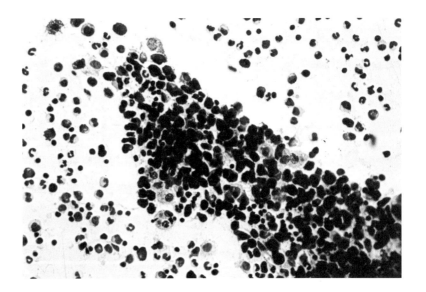

5
Disorders of lymphocytes

5.1. Pertussis (whooping cough)
Blood film

Typical haematological findings in pertussis include a very high lymphocytosis which may reach $100 \times 10^9/l$. In addition, the cells may have prominent nucleoli and basophilic cytoplasm as shown in this high-power view. The film appearance can be mistaken for lymphoblastic leukaemia.

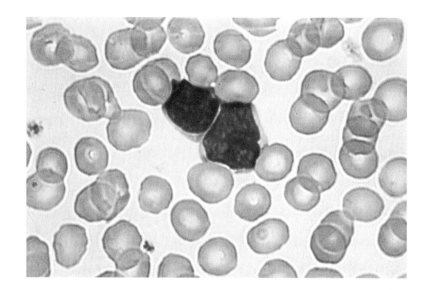

5.2. Infectious mononucleosis
Blood film

Infection with circulating EB virus causes a preponderance (more than 25 per cent) of circulating 'atypical mononuclear' cells which are mostly activated T lymphocytes. Morphologically they have basophilic cytoplasm displaying characteristic darker 'crimped' areas where they impinge upon red cells. Nucleoli are often prominent and distinction of these cells from leukaemic blasts can sometimes be very difficult.

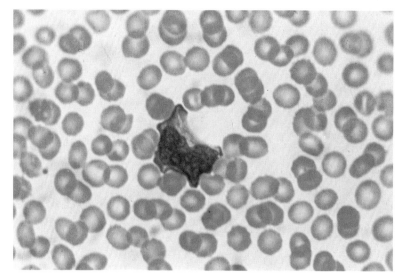

5.3. Infectious mononucleosis
Blood film
This plate shows another 'activated' lymphocyte with less prominent nucleoli than that shown in 5.2.

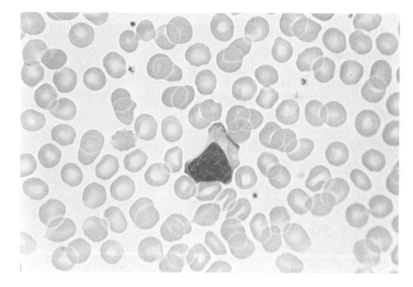

5.4. Persistent CMV infection
Blood film
Cytomegalovirus is another agent producing an infectious mononucleosis-like syndrome (compare 5.2 and 5.3). This plate shows a preponderance of mature lymphocytes with hypochromic red cells. This two-year-old boy had a persistent infection and later developed abdominal lymphoma.

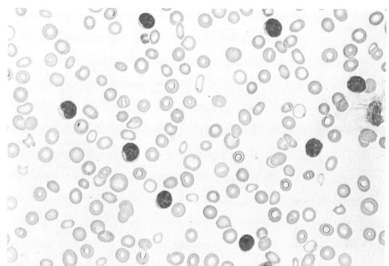

5.5. Persistent CMV infection
Blood film
The same patient's blood as shown in 5.4 again demonstrates a 'mature' lymphocytosis but some activated cells with basophilic cytoplasm are also seen.

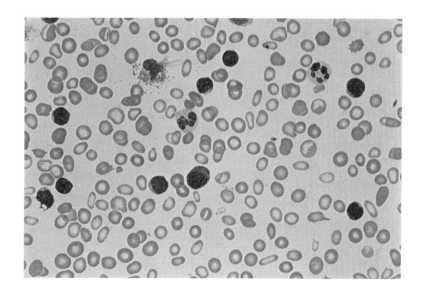

5.6. CMV infection
Blood film

These atypical lymphocytes show how
CMV can be confused with infectious
mononucleosis and even acute leukaemia,
although the proportion of atypical forms is
usually less than 25 per cent.

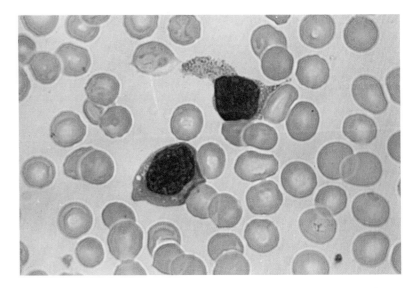

5.7. CMV infection in a 12-month-old infant
Bone marrow

The marrow shows 20 per cent
lymphoblasts and 35 per cent lymphocytes
and could easily be mistaken for
leukaemia. CMV was cultured from the
urine, throat, and blood buffy coat.

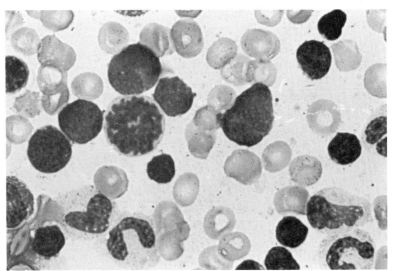

6
Platelet disorders

6.1. Idiopathic thrombocytopenic purpura (ITP)
Bone marrow

Large numbers of apparently immature and non-budding megakaryocytes are present. Although plentiful megakaryocytes are always seen in ITP, suggesting peripheral destruction of platelets, the morphological features are not diagnostic.

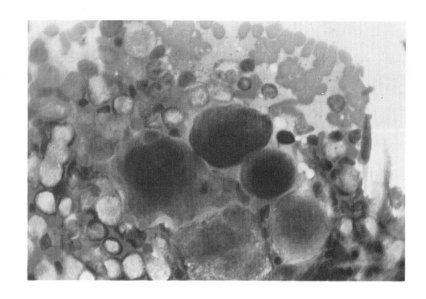

6.2. Bernard–Soulier syndrome
Blood film

This, along with the May–Hegglin anomaly and other rarer syndromes, e.g. that associated with nephritis and deafness, is one of the 'giant platelet' disorders. Inheritance is autosomal and incompletely recessive. As shown here, the platelets are almost as large as red cells. The long bleeding time in this condition results from the platelets' lack of a receptor site for Factor VIII associated protein (VIII^{Rag}).

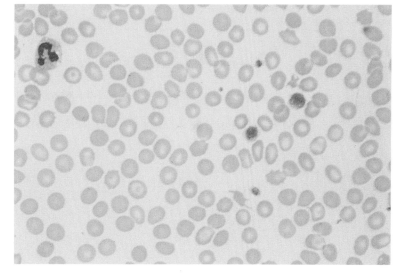

6.3. Bernard–Soulier syndrome
Blood film

Splenectomy was performed in this patient and a Howell–Jolly body is shown along with giant platelets. In fact, neither splenectomy nor corticosteroids are of clinical benefit.

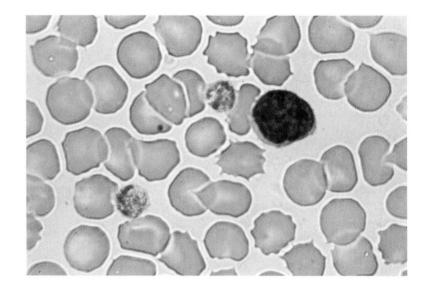

6.4. Bernard–Soulier syndrome
Blood film: electron micrograph, × 5900

In this preparation the platelets can be seen to be almost equal in size to the white blood cells.

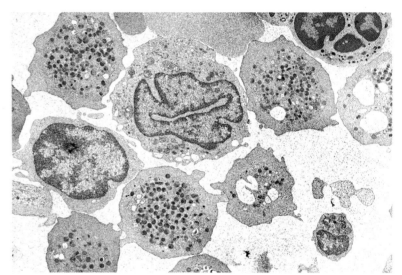

6.5. May–Hegglin anomaly
Blood film

Inheritance of this disorder is autosomal dominant and one-third of patients are thrombocytopenic. Neutrophil inclusions are present and resemble the Döhle bodies found in infected patients. The neutrophils show a 'sausage' shape of their nuclear lobes and giant platelets also occur.

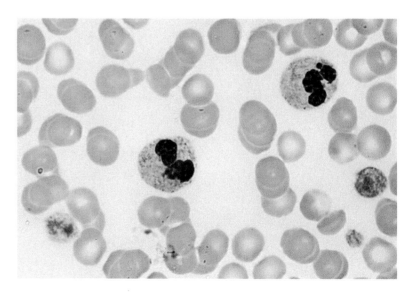

6.6. Wiskott–Aldrich syndrome
Blood film
Chronic thrombocytopenia, susceptibility to infection, and eczema characterize this sex-linked recessive disorder. The associated immunodeficiency is characterized by humoral and cellular abnormalities and susceptibility to lymphoreticular malignancies. This plate shows thrombocytopenia with typical very small platelets.

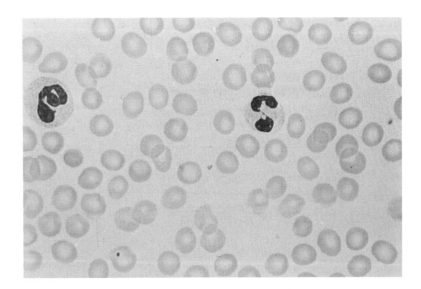

6.7. Thrombocytosis
Blood film
The platelet count in this blood sample was $1 \times 10^{12}/1$. There is marked anisothrombia. This patient had a reactive thrombocytosis following bleeding from a Meckel's diverticulum. Differential diagnosis is from: hyposplenism; infection; renal disease; myeloproliferative disorders; and other causes of marrow regeneration.

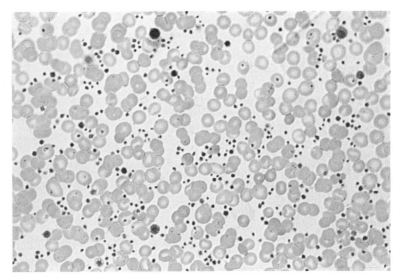

6.8. Gray platelet syndrome
Blood film
The patient presented with mild thrombocytopenia, mild bleeding problems and large agranular blue-gray platelets in the blood. Platelet aggregation is impaired but nucleotide and serotonin levels are normal. There is a profound abnormality in granule formation and a deficiency in α-granule substances, e.g. fibrinogen, β-thromboglobulin, platelet factor 4, coagulation factor V and growth-promoting factor.

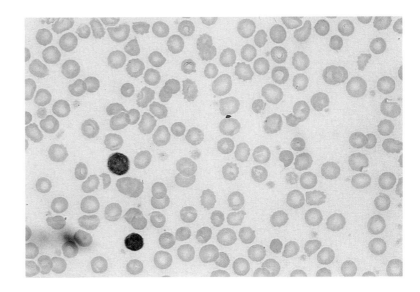

6.9. Electron micrograph of normal platelets
Blood

Normal platelets, seen here, contain dense bodies (few), which are not found in every platelet, α-granules, which are numerous and present in all platelets, as well as endoplasmic reticulum and mitochondria.

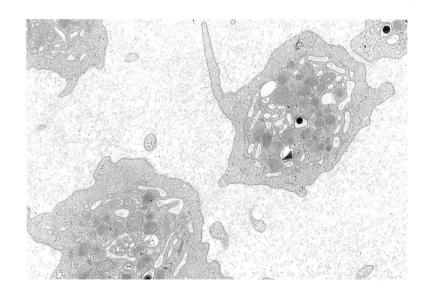

6.10. Electron micrograph of Gray platelets
Blood

The platelets in this disorder lack the α-granules of the normal, but otherwise the complement of organelles is normal. The lack of α-granules gives rise to the pale gray staining in routine blood films.

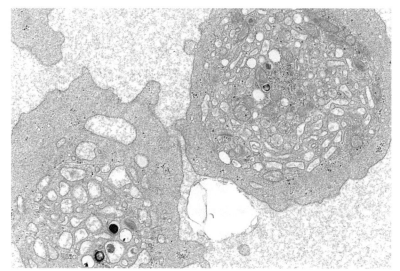

7
Acute Lymphoblastic Leukaemia (ALL)

7.1. ALL FAB type L1
Bone marrow

The most frequent type of childhood leukaemia, the blasts are small and lymphocytoid. There is a high nuclear:cytoplasmic ratio and nucleoli are generally not visible. L1 morphology is seen in all immunologically defined ALL subtypes except B-ALL, most commonly it is associated with CD10 positivity, with or without cytoplasmic immunoglobulin. Hyperdiploidy (>50 chromosomes) is also more common in L1 disease.

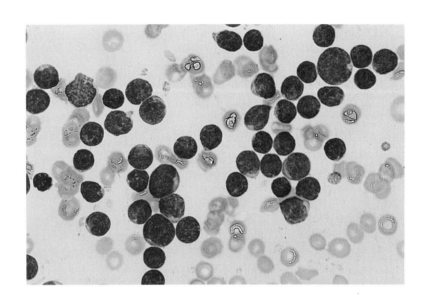

7.2. ALL FAB type L1 with vacuoles
Bone marrow

Vacuoles are found in the blasts from around 25 per cent of cases of childhood ALL. They are not confined to the L3 subtype. They are associated with periodic acid-Schiff positivity, CD10 positivity and a low circulating white cell count. Patients in this group have a prognostic advantage. Vacuoles are occasionally seen in L2 disease.

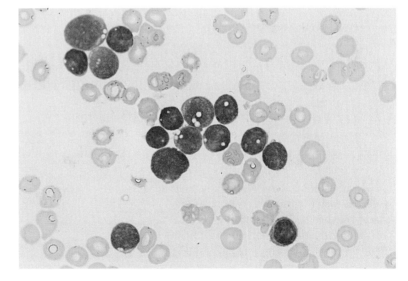

7.3. ALL FAB type L1 with 'hand mirror' cells
Bone marrow

The curious but striking amoeboid configuration of blast cells in some leukaemias has been likened to a hand mirror. The significance, if any, of this is unclear. Conflicting claims for prognostic significance have been made, though more have suggested it to be an adverse feature. The frequency of cases with >10 per cent hand mirrors is low, below 5 per cent. They are not confined to L1 ALL.

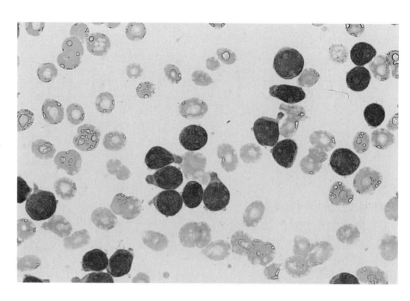

7.4. ALL FAB type L1 with granules
Bone marrow

Up to 7 per cent of cases of ALL will show conspicuous peroxidase-negative azurophilic granules, the nature and importance of which are presently unknown.

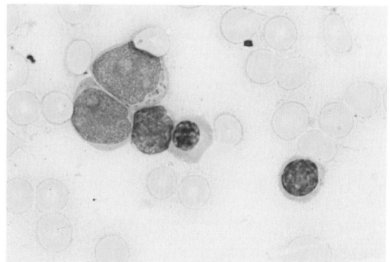

7.5. ALL FAB type L2
Bone marrow

L2 ALL accounts for 10–15 per cent of all cases and is defined by the presence of a low nuclear:cytoplasmic ratio, conspicuous nucleoli, irregular nuclear outlines, and bigger blast cells. It is associated with periodic acid-Schiff negativity, and arises more often in older children. L2 disease is more resistant to treatment.

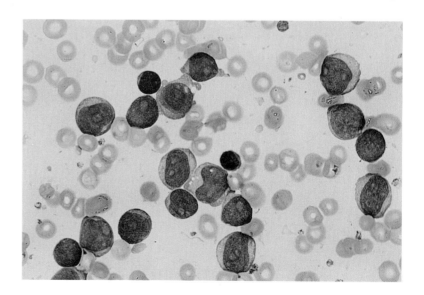

7.6. ALL FAB type L2
Bone marrow
Another example to show variable
morphology (see 7.5).

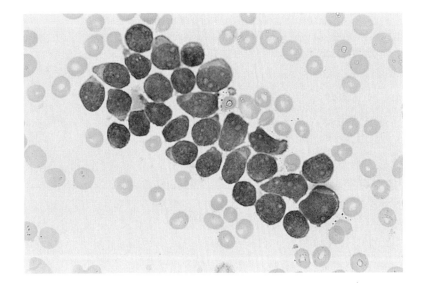

7.7. ALL FAB type L3
Bone marrow
The rarest type of ALL, L3 accounts for
<1 per cent of cases. It is nearly always of
B-cell immunophenotype, a type which
does not arise in L1 or L2 disease. The cells
are large, densely basophilic, heavily
vacuolated and variably have conspicuous
nucleoli. It is associated with a non-random
chromosome abnormality (t(8;14)). The
vacuoles are usually positive for oil red O.

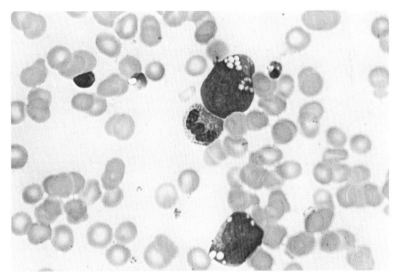

7.8. ALL FAB type L3
Bone marrow
A further example (see 7.7). While the
morphology is usually unequivocal,
confusion with other FAB types can occur.

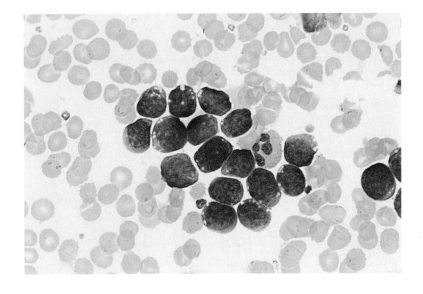

7.9. ALL cytochemistry

Bone marrow; PAS reaction
Periodic acid-Schiff (PAS) positivity in
'blocks' and coarse granules is commonly
found in childhood ALL—between 50 and
60 per cent of cases. Vacuoles (other than
in L3 disease) are associated with
positivity, as is CD10 reactivity, a low
white count and L1 morphology. L2 disease
is more often negative. PAS positive
disease thus associates with good
prognostic features.

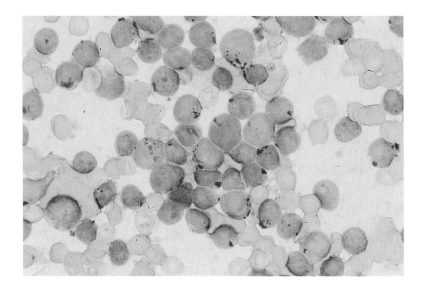

7.10. ALL cytochemistry

Bone marrow; acid phosphatase
Non-diffuse acid phosphatase positivity is
found typically in T-cell ALL as in this
case. It is not exclusively so, being negative
in 5–10 per cent of T-cell cases and positive
in a third of non-T diseases. Positivity in
non-T ALL is usually much weaker than in
T-ALL, but not invariably.

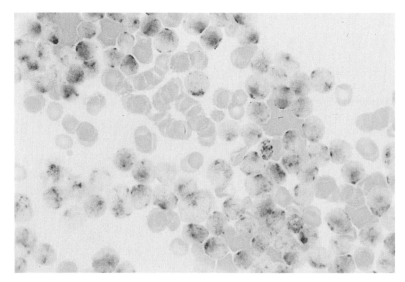

7.11. ALL cytochemistry

Bone marrow; oil red O
Lymphoblasts, particularly the heavily
vacuolated L3 type (though not
exclusively so), take up the lipid stain oil
red O. The stain is seldom helpful in
distinguishing subtypes of ALL, or in
distinguishing ALL from other leukaemias.

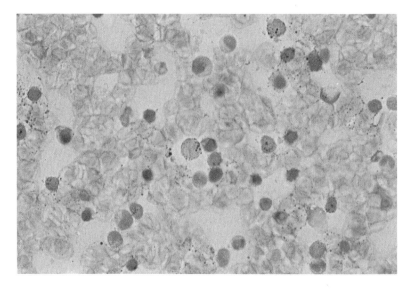

7.12. ALL marrow histology

Trephine biopsy; HE stain
Diffuse total marrow replacement with loss of fat spaces is the commonest finding in childhood ALL.

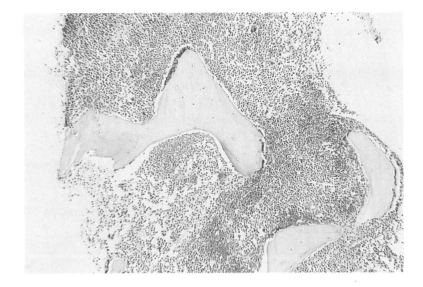

7.13. ALL marrow histology

Trephine biopsy; reticulin stain
Around 10–20 per cent of cases have sufficient secondary marrow fibrosis to make aspiration very difficult.

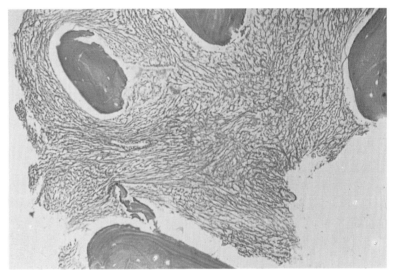

7.14. ALL marrow histology

Trephine biopsy; HE stain
Patchy infiltration with preservation of normal architecture is sometimes seen in the so-called 'lymphoma–leukaemia' syndrome, typical of T-cell ALL as in this case.

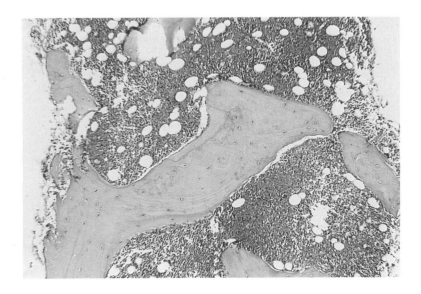

7.15. Extramedullary ALL—CNS
Cytocentrifuge preparation; cerebrospinal fluid

CNS leukaemia as an isolated relapse; cell count $0.1 \times 10^9/l$. The morphology may be distorted in such preparations and appear different from that seen in blood or marrow smears.

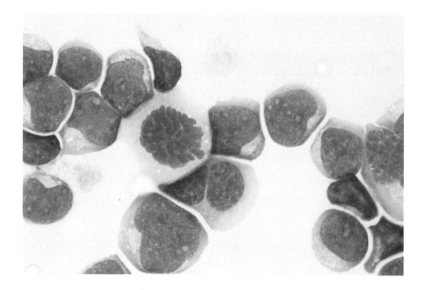

7.16. Extramedullary ALL—CNS
Cytocentrifuge preparation; cerebrospinal fluid

CNS leukaemia as part of a multi-site relapse. Cell count $2 \times 10^9/l$.

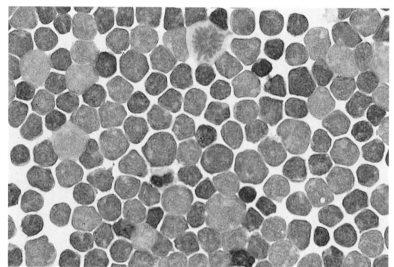

7.17. Extramedullary ALL—CNS
Paraffin section of superficial cerebral cortex post mortem; HE stain

Dense meningeal infiltration extending down the intracerebral perivascular meningeal sheaths but no direct invasion of brain tissue. Even in advanced disease direct neural invasion is unusual.

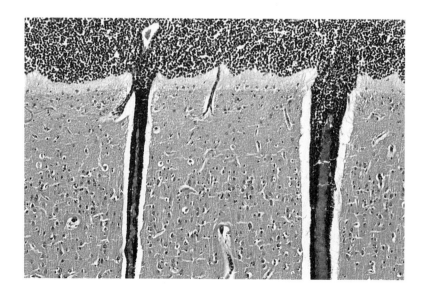

7.18. Extramedullary ALL—pleural effusion

Cytocentrifuge preparation; pleural fluid

A malignant pleural effusion in T-ALL. Such effusions are more frequent in the 'leukaemia–lymphoma' syndrome typical of T-ALL and B-ALL.

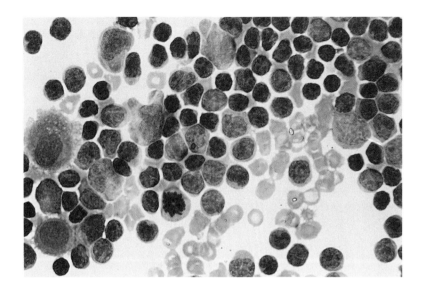

7.19. Extramedullary ALL—anterior chamber of eye

Microneedle aspirate of anterior chamber

On rare occasions this complication can be an isolated phenomenon without evidence of disease elsewhere. It can be the sole site of detectable active disease.

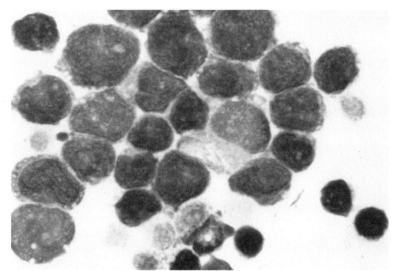

7.20. Extramedullary ALL— testicular infiltration

Paraffin section; HE stain

A common site of isolated late relapse. The section shows a light interstitial infiltrate between the seminiferous tubules in an elective biopsy done at the end of treatment in a boy thought to be in complete remission.

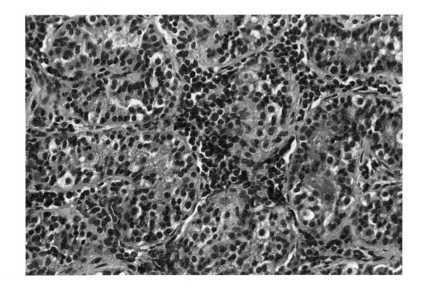

7.21. Biphenotypic relapse of ALL
Bone marrow

Rarely relapse of ALL may show features of both ALL and AML. There can be two populations evident morphologically as in this case.

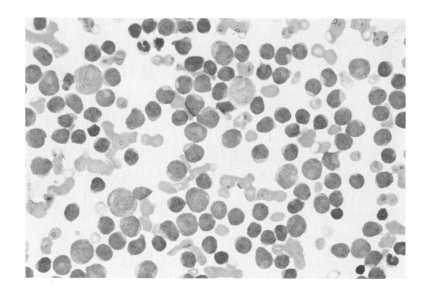

7.22. ALL; 'rebound' lymphocytosis
Bone marrow (low power)

Extreme degrees of lymphocytosis with an excess of blasts are very common in patients who have recently stopped chemotherapy. It cannot be emphasized strongly enough that mistakes in marrow interpretation are frequently made at this stage and extreme caution must *always* be exercised.

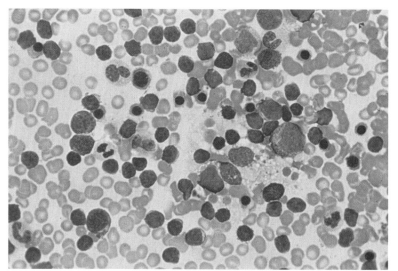

7.23. ALL; 'rebound' lymphocytosis
Bone marrow (high power)

A high-power view of the patient's marrow shown in 7.22 shows the presence of a lymphoblast and a number of lymphocytes. This phenomenon can persist for over a year and has no demonstrable prognostic significance. These 'normal' blasts are terminal deoxynucleotidyl transferase-positive and bear surface 'common ALL antigen'.

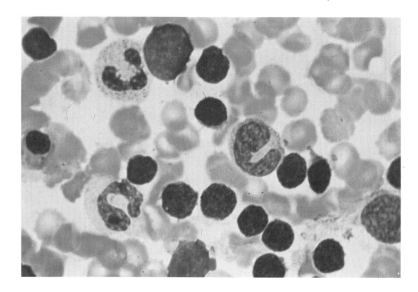

8
Acute non-lymphoblastic leukaemia

8.1. Acute myeloid leukaemia FAB type M1
Bone marrow

Chiefly type 1 (agranular) blasts. Differentiation from ALL type L2 on Romanowsky-stained morphology can be difficult; the latter is more common.

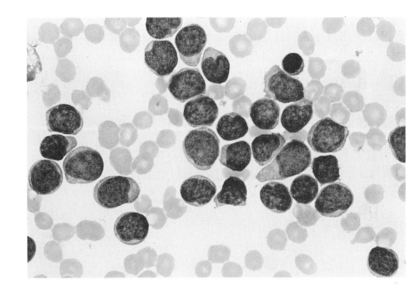

8.2. Acute myeloid leukaemia FAB type M1
Bone marrow; peroxidase stain

Same case as 8.1; 2–3 per cent cells show positivity, one with a splinter-like Auer rod.

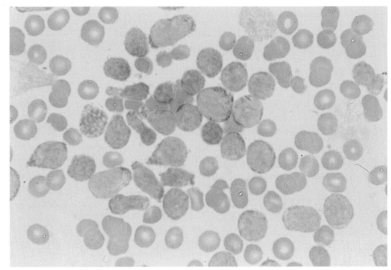

8.3. Acute myeloid leukaemia FAB type M2

Bone marrow

Distinguished from M1 by a greater proportion of type 2 (granular) blasts easily seen on Romanowsky staining. Auer rods, as in this case, often visible. Blasts may show a t(8; 21) karyotype.

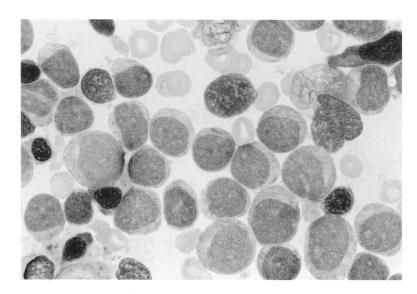

8.4. Acute myeloid leukaemia FAB type M2

Bone marrow

High-power view of an Auer rod.

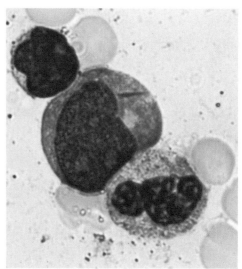

8.5. Acute myeloid leukaemia FAB type M2

Bone marrow; peroxidase stain

A greater proportion of cells staining with greater intensity than in type M1 (8.2). Auer rods appear thicker showing intense peroxidase activity.

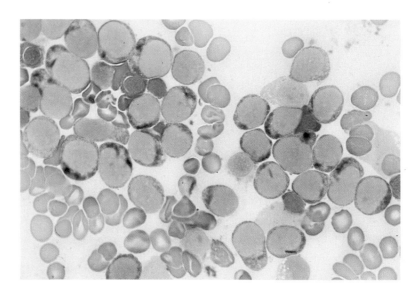

8.6. Acute myeloid leukaemia FAB type M2

Bone marrow; Sudan black stain
Peroxidase and Sudan black stains closely correlate with each other.

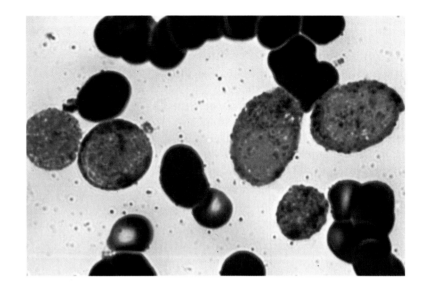

8.7. Acute myeloid leukaemia FAB type M3

Bone marrow
Promyelocytic leukaemia. Dense azurophil granules fill the cytoplasm. The nucleus shows variable shape and site within the cell. Such cells are strongly peroxidase positive and sudanophilic.
Characteristically has a t(15; 17) karyotype.

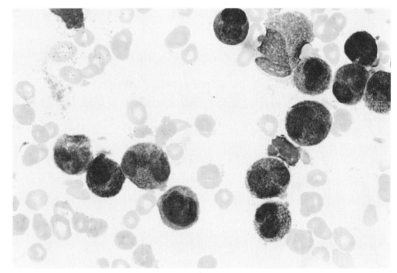

8.8. Acute myeloid leukaemia FAB type M3

Blood film
A high-power view of a malignant promyelocyte showing numerous Auer rods—the so-called 'faggot' cell.

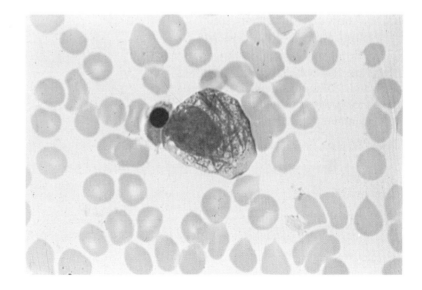

8.9. Acute myeloid leukaemia M3 variant
Blood film

A hypogranular variant of M3 is recognized which, like the typical variety, can cause a consumption coagulopathy, but where the cells are not so strikingly granular. It also shows the t(15; 17) karyotype. The cells show nuclear convolution and are mostly not heavily granulated, but there are a few 'faggot' cells to be found.

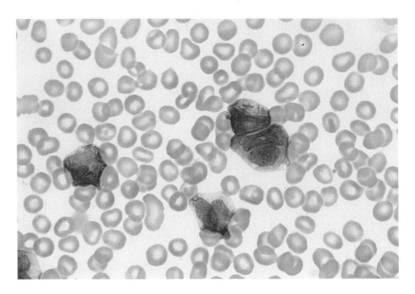

8.10. Acute myelomonocytic leukaemia (AMML)—FAB type M4
Blood film

M4 AMML is defined by 20–80 per cent non-erythroid cells in the marrow being monocyte-related and (typically) the circulating monoblast/monocyte count being $>5 \times 10^9/l$.

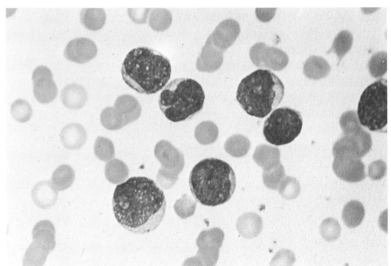

8.11. Acute myelomonocytic leukaemia—FAB type M4
Bone marrow

Blasts are >30 per cent of non-erythroid cells, and >20 per cent but <80 per cent show monocytic features (cytochemically and/or immunologically).

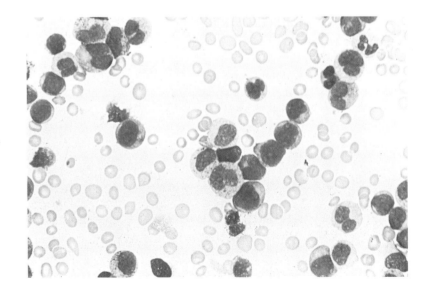

8.12. Acute myelomonocytic leukaemia—FAB type M4
Bone marrow; combined esterase stain

Combined chloroacetate and α-naphthyl acetate esterase stain with fast blue BB for coupling the former and hexazonium pararosanilin for the latter. The monocytic (brown) component is admixed with the granulocyte (blue) component.

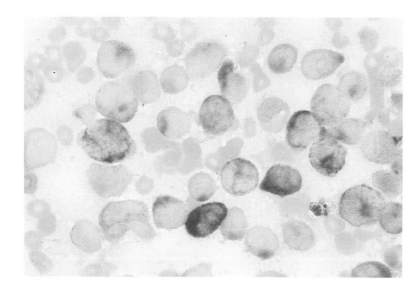

8.13. Acute myelomonocytic leukaemia with eosinophils
Bone marrow

The presence of numerous atypical eosinophils marks this variant of M4 AMML which is also associated with a specific chromosome abnormality (inv/del (16) (q22)).

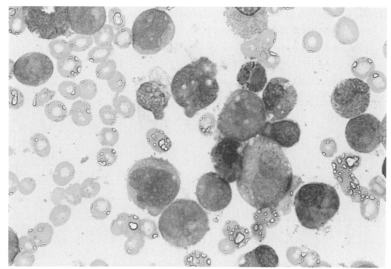

8.14. Acute monocytic leukaemia (AMoL)—FAB type M5
Bone marrow

Over 80 per cent of blasts show monocytic lineage, cytochemically and immunologically. Romanowsky morphology is hard to distinguish in some cases from M1 or L2.

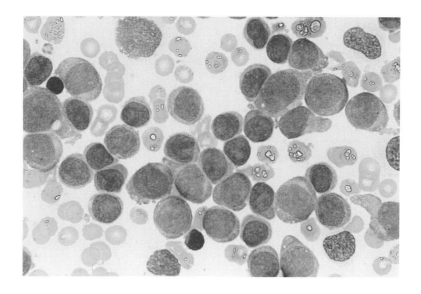

8.15. Acute monocytic leukaemia
Bone marrow; combined
esterase stain

The same case as 8.14 stained as in 8.12.
There are no chloroacetate esterase-
positive cells present—only those with
α-naphthyl acetate esterase.

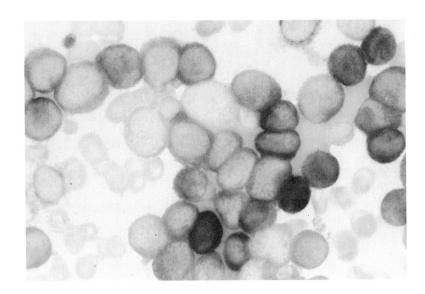

8.16. Acute monocytic leukaemia
with erythrophagocytosis
Bone marrow

A variant of M5 AMoL that is
characterized by erythrophagocytosis and
a specific chromosome abnormality
(t(8; 16)(p11; p13)).

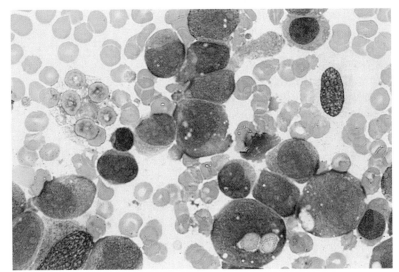

8.17. Acute erythroleukaemia
(AEL)—FAB type M6
Bone marrow

Criteria for this diagnosis include: >30 per
cent of non-erythroid cells are type 1 or 2
blast cells (see 8.1 and 8.3); >50 per cent
of all cells are erythroid. This category of
disease is very rare in childhood. The
photograph is of the disease in a 15-year-
old.

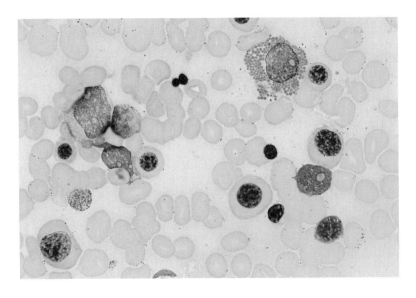

8.18. Acute erythroleukaemia
Blood film; PAS reaction
Erythroblasts in M6 AEL show coarse or diffuse variable to strong periodic acid-Schiff (PAS) positivity in around 50 per cent of cases.

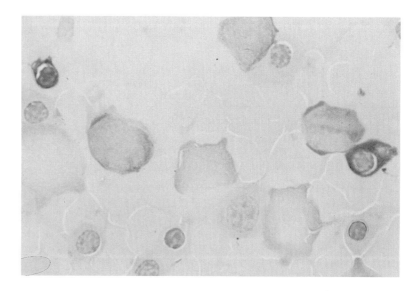

8.19. Acute megakaryoblastic leukaemia (AMKL)—FAB type M7
Bone marrow
AMKL cannot be diagnosed on morphology alone, and requires the demonstration of platelet peroxidase on electron microscopy or antigens recognized by platelet or factor VIII-specific mono- or polyclonal antibodies. Cytochemical patterns vary: there may be non-diffuse α-naphthyl acetate esterase and/or acid phosphatase. Blasts vary in size and may have cytoplasmic blebs as in the case illustrated. The disease is rare in normal children, but is seen more frequently in those with Down's syndrome. Chromosome 21 may be abnormal in M7 blasts from non-Down's children.

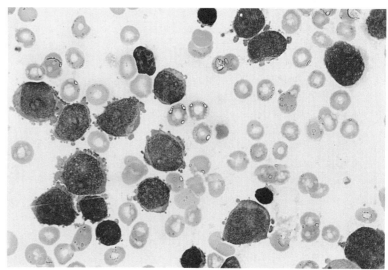

8.20. Acute megakaryoblastic leukaemia—marrow fibrosis
Trephine biopsy; reticulin stain
Associated secondary marrow fibrosis is a common feature of M7 AMKL and may make aspiration extremely difficult.

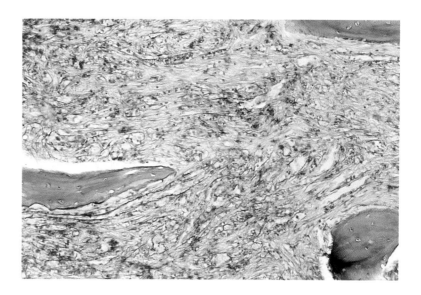

8.21. Acute megakaryoblastic leukaemia—platelet glycoprotein expression
Bone marrow
Alkaline phosphatase anti-alkaline phosphatase (APAAP) technique showing strong positivity for CDw42 (Gp1b) in a patient with M7 AML.

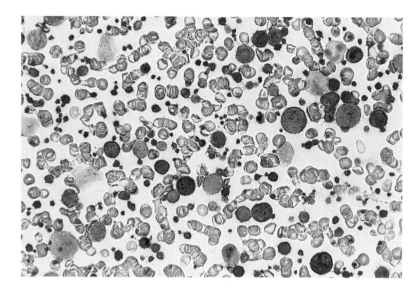

8.22. Acute megakaryoblastic leukaemia—factor VIII antigen expression
Trephine biopsy
Immunoperoxidase staining of factor VIII antigen in blasts in a section of marrow from a child with AMKL.

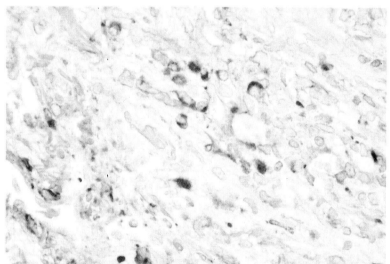

8.23. Acute myeloid leukaemia; CNS relapse
CSF cytocentrifuge
CNS relapse does occur in AML and can be diagnosed on a cytocentrifuge preparation from CSF. Numerous myeloblasts and some monocytes are seen.

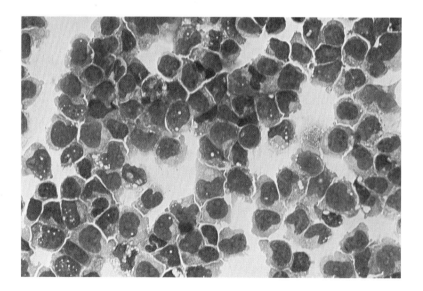

8.24. Acute myeloid leukaemia—CNS relapse
CSF cytocentrifuge

A further example from an infant with congenital leukaemia (type M5).

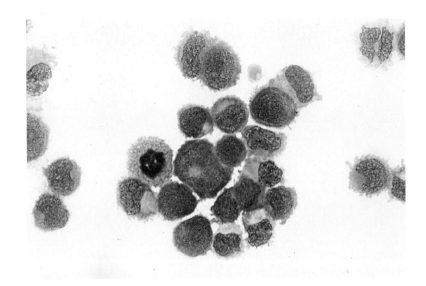

8.25. CGL myeloid blast crisis
Blood film

The chronic phase of CGL often terminates as 'blast crisis'—either lymphoid, myeloid, or mixed. This particular girl presented with a myeloid blast crisis 5 years from diagnosis. Many myeloblasts are present along with other abnormal myeloid precursors including degranulated basophils and eosinophils.

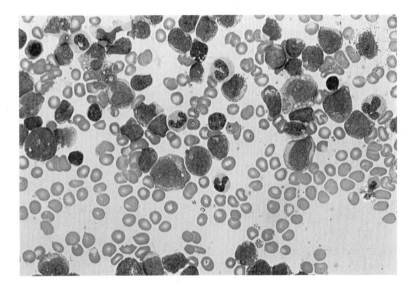

9
Myeloproliferative disorders

9.1. Down's syndrome—leukaemoid reaction
Blood film
Film from three-day-old simple trisomy Down's syndrome baby showing blast cells. His WBC was 44 × 10^9/l (37 per cent blasts); haemoglobin 24.7 g/dl; platelets 120 × 10^9/l. The marrow is shown in 9.2. The blasts disappeared by the age of three months and bone marrow failure never occurred. The boy remains well 5 years later.

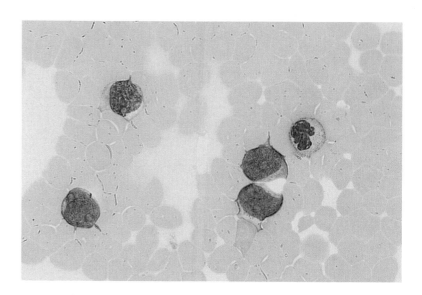

9.2. Down's syndrome—leukaemoid reaction
Bone marrow
Marrow aspirate from same case as 9.1 concurrent with blood film. Blasts comprised only 18 per cent of the total nucleated cells. Karyotype on bone marrow showed simple trisomy 21. The blasts appeared myeloid in origin. No megakaryocyte markers were assessed.

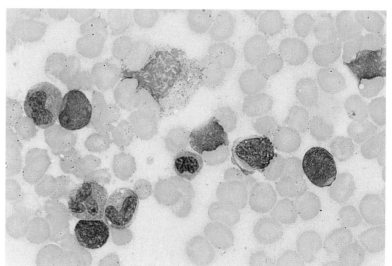

9.3. Down's syndrome—leukaemoid reaction
Trephine biopsy
Concurrent with 9.1 and 9.2 from same case. Heterogeneous cell population with no evidence of leukaemia. Cellularity unremarkable for age.

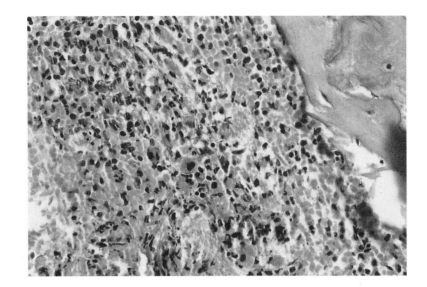

9.4. Down's syndrome—myelofibrosis/leukaemia; RAEB(T)
Blood film
Circulating blasts in a 3½-year-old simple trisomy Down syndrome girl. She had had a perinatal leukaemoid phase as above (9.1, 9.2, 9.3) with a WBC of 169 × 10⁹/l, aged four days, which disappeared without marrow failure over two months. The blasts marked with CDw41 (platelet glycoprotein IIb/IIIa). They reappeared three years later with progressive marrow failure and fibrosis. Haemoglobin 6.6 g/dl; WBC 30.9 × 10⁹/l; blasts 8 per cent, platelets 64 × 10⁹/l.

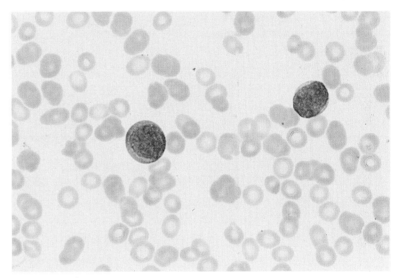

9.5. Down's syndrome—myelofibrosis/leukaemia; RAEB(T)
Bone marrow
Same case as 9.4. Marrow very difficult to aspirate; blasts 25 per cent of nucleated cells. Karyotype of marrow showed mosaicism with most cells having abnormalities additional to the trisomy 21 (48, XX, 6q−, +11, +21). Blasts appeared to be of megakaryocyte lineage. Two are seen in this frame. At this stage the syndrome would qualify for the group of myelodysplasias known as RAEB(T).

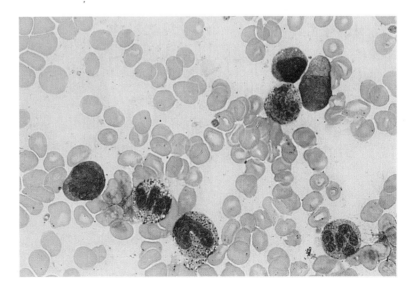

9.6. Down's syndrome—
myelofibrosis/leukaemia;
RAEB(T)
Trephine biopsy
Low power view showing gross
hypercellularity. Same case as 9.4.

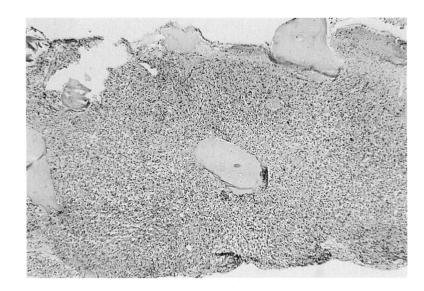

9.7. Down's syndrome—
myelofibrosis/leukaemia;
RAEB(T)
Trephine biopsy; reticulin stain
Increased reticulin and fibroblasts (same
case as 9.4).

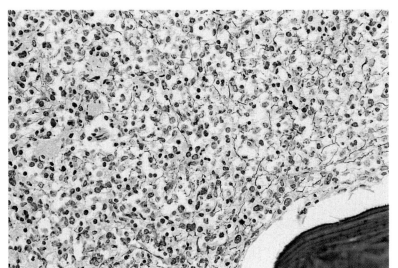

9.8. RAEB(T)
Bone marrow
A six-year-old girl with a pancytopenia and
a few circulating blast cells and myelocytes.
A rare condition in childhood without
monosomy 7 (see below), which usually
progresses to acute leukaemia.

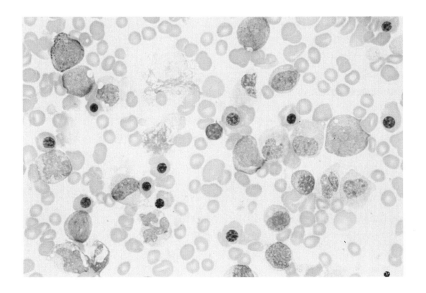

9.9. RAEB with monosomy 7
Blood film

A childhood syndrome characterized by hepatosplenomegaly, recurrent infections, myeloproliferation and refractory anaemia with a variable excess of blasts. It can be distinguished from juvenile chronic myelomonocytic leukaemia (see below) by the chromosome abnormality and lack of fetal red cell changes. The patient illustrated had a high WBC which tends to evolve as the disease progresses. The eventual transformation to acute myeloid leukaemia is the rule. The tendency to infection is at least in part due to an associated neutrophil function defect.

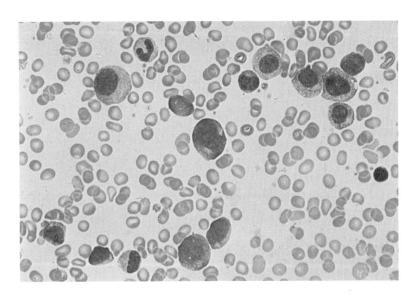

9.10. RAEB with monosomy 7
Bone marrow

An excess of blasts (8 per cent in this aspirate) with associated erythrodysplasia.

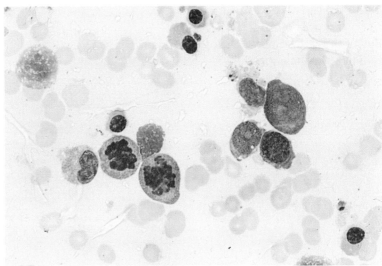

9.11. RAEB with monosomy 7
Bone marrow

As above; atypical and poorly granulated myeloid precursors.

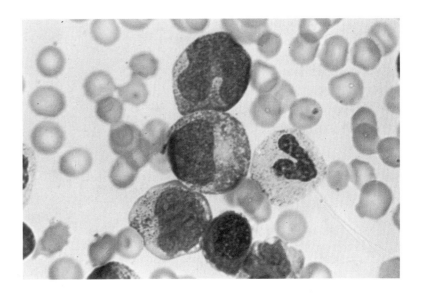

9.12. RAEB with monosomy 7
Bone marrow
As above; eosinophils with atypical morphology are commonly seen.

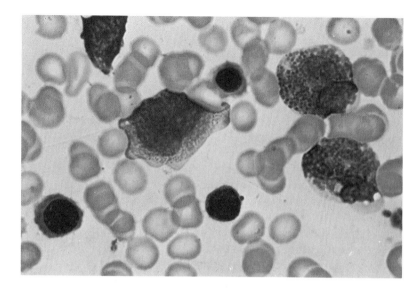

9.13. RAEB with monosomy 7
Trephine biopsy
Boy of five years. Shows myeloproliferation with mixed population.

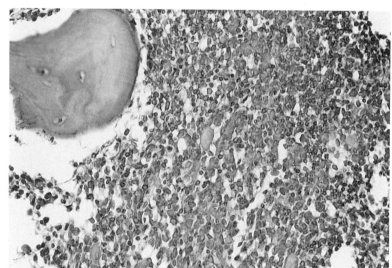

9.14. RAEB with monosomy 7
Trephine biopsy; reticulin stain
Increased reticulin and accompanying fibrosis are usual in this syndrome—aspiration of marrow is often difficult.

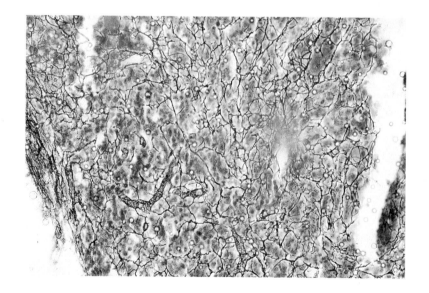

9.15. Juvenile chronic myeloid leukaemia (JCML)
Blood film

This condition is more accurately called childhood subacute myelomonocytic leukaemia. It arises in infants and can be distinguished from 'adult' type chronic granulocytic leukaemia (see below) by the clinical picture (lymphadenopathy, skin rashes, bruising); the blood findings (fetal red cell characteristics, thrombocytopenia, atypical monocytosis) and marrow cytogenetics (the Ph[1] chromosome is absent). Otherwise the two disorders can be confused. In the child illustrated, the WBC was $18 \times 10^9/l$ with 17 per cent monocytes with the morphology shown.

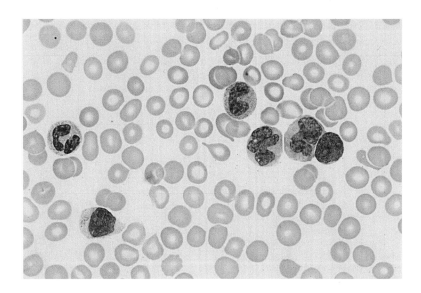

9.16. Juvenile chronic myeloid leukaemia
Bone marrow

A mixed picture with a variable though usually modest excess of blasts.

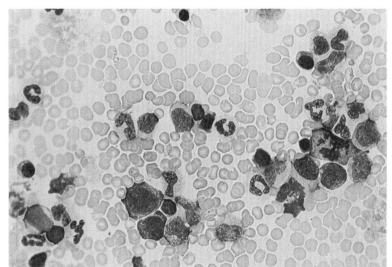

9.17. Juvenile chronic myeloid leukaemia
Bone marrow

Abnormal eosinophils are frequently seen in the bone marrow and blood. These may be degranulated or, as shown here, contain large vacuoles.

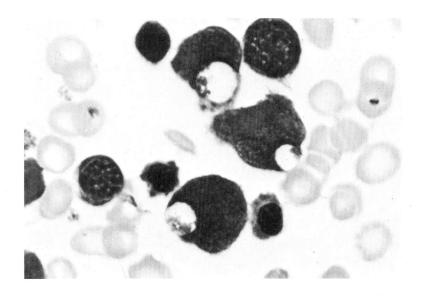

9.18. Juvenile chronic myeloid leukaemia
Trephine biopsy
Dense hypercellular marrow. Child aged three.

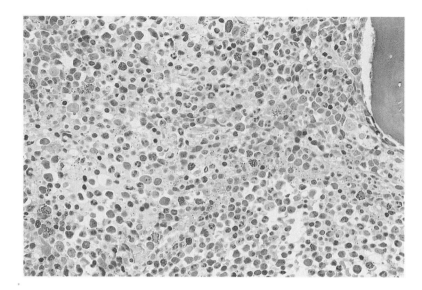

9.19. Juvenile chronic myeloid leukaemia
Blood film; Kleihauer stain
A striking characteristic of JCML is the frequently encountered high concentration of HbF with a heterogeneous distribution among the red cells as shown in this untransfused patient. Parallel fetal red cell changes seen include increased i antigen expression, and reduced carbonic anhydrase. Such features are not invariable.

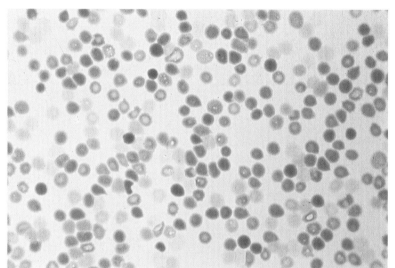

9.20. 'Adult' type chronic granulocytic leukaemia
Blood film
The disease seen in children does not differ from that seen in adults. The presenting features are similar—massive splenomegaly, gross leucocytosis sometimes sufficient to cause vascular sludging, (in the case illustrated, a 10-year-old boy, the WBC was $849 \times 10^9/l$) anaemia and fatigue. There is usually an associated basophilia, and granulocyte alkaline phosphatase activity is low. The Ph[1] chromosome is nearly always present.

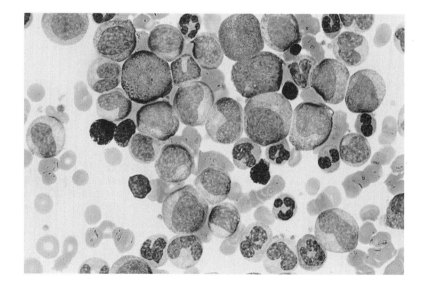

9.21. 'Adult' type chronic granulocytic leukaemia
Bone marrow
Cytology of marrow aspirates is not qualitatively abnormal in any specific way. There is little associated fibrosis, so a densely cellular aspirate is usually easily obtained.

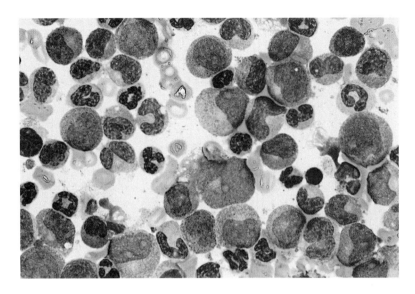

9.22. 'Adult' type chronic granulocytic leukaemia
Bone marrow
Foam cells (macrophages) and cells resembling Gaucher cells are sometimes seen in the marrow giving rise to a mistaken diagnosis of a storage disorder (see 9.23).

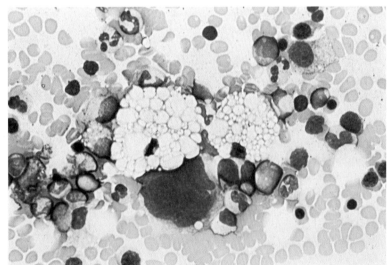

9.23. 'Adult' type chronic granulocytic leukaemia
Bone marrow
Pseudo–Gaucher cells (see 9.22).

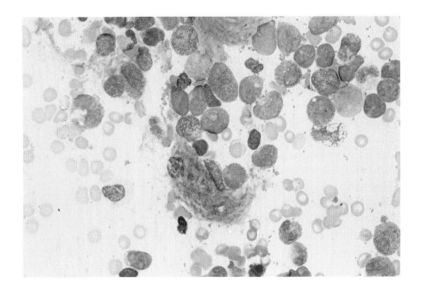

9.24. 'Adult' type chronic granulocytic leukaemia
Trephine biopsy
Myeloproliferation with total loss of fat spaces (same patient as 9.20, 9.21).

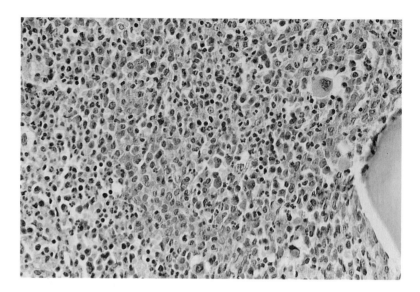

9.25. 'Adult' type chronic granulocytic leukaemia—Ph¹ negative
Blood film
Occasional examples of Ph[1] negative CGL (other than juvenile CML) are seen in childhood. This film is from a nine-year-old whose disease was clinically more aggressive than Ph[1] positive CGL. She responded well to a histocompatible marrow allograft.

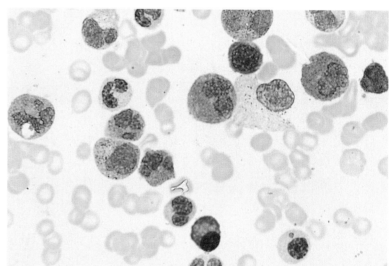

9.26. Primary myelofibrosis
Blood film
Primary myelofibrosis (agnogenic myeloid metaplasia, AMM) is an adult disorder that is very rare in childhood and any patient who might have it should be thoroughly investigated to exclude other causes of marrow fibrosis such as those above. It does occur. The patient illustrated had concomitant folate lack, which can complicate any myeloproliferative state. Tear-drop poikilocytes are seen in the case illustrated. Other features include leucoerythroblastosis, Pelger–Hüet cells and giant platelets.

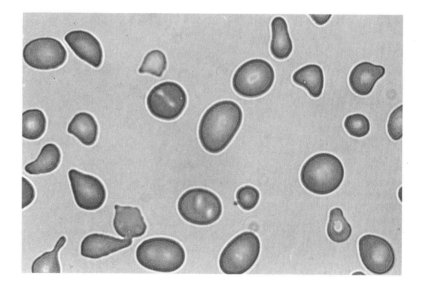

9.27. Primary myelofibrosis
Trephine biopsy; reticulin stain
This shows the typical fibrillary pattern of a myelofibrotic marrow and is taken from the patient whose blood film is shown in 9.26.

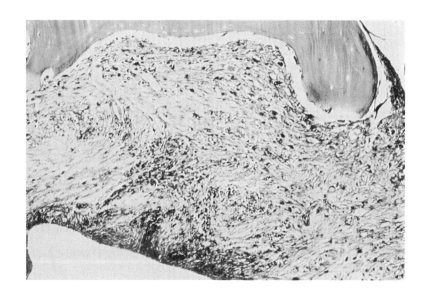

10
Histiomonocytic disorders

Classification of histiocytosis syndromes
    (after Histiocyte Society Classification; *Lancet* (1987). 1, 208–9)

1. **Langerhans cell histiocytosis** (formerly eosinophilic granuloma, Hand–Schüller–Christian disease, Letterer–Siwe disease)

2. **Histiocytoses of mononuclear phagocytes other than Langerhans cells:**
    (a)   familial erythrophagocytic lymphohistiocytosis
    (b)   sporadic erythrophagocytic lymphohistiocytosis
    (c)   infection-associated haemophagocytic syndrome
    (d)   Rosai Dorfman disease
    (e)   xanthogranuloma
    (f)   reticulohistiocytoma

3. **Malignant histiocytic disorders:**
    (a)   monocytic leukaemia
    (b)   malignant histiocytosis
    (c)   true histiocytic lymphoma

10.1. Langerhans cell histiocytosis
Bone marrow

This two-year-old boy had marked hepatosplenomegaly, disseminated bone disease and a skin rash. The changes in the bone marrow are very variable and are generally not diagnostic. In some cases large foamy histiocytes are found in the marrow aspirate. In other instances the histiocytes may be less mature looking and can resemble those found in the skin lesions. There is no general agreement about the prognostic importance of these appearances.

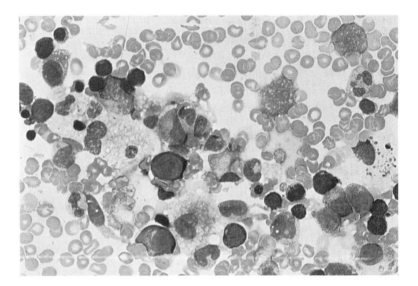

10.2. Langerhans cell histiocytosis
Bone marrow trephine; plastic section

The morphology of the cells is better seen than in paraffin sections and the typical folded nucleus and reniform nuclear shapes are readily appreciated.

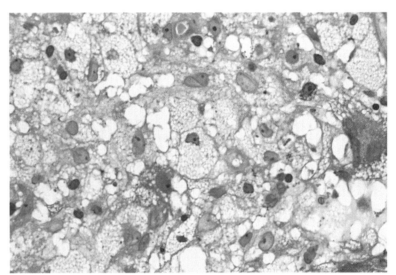

10.3. Langerhans cell histiocytosis
Bone marrow

Here the marrow contained many cells with long processes. This appearance is striking but is not diagnostic without marker studies.

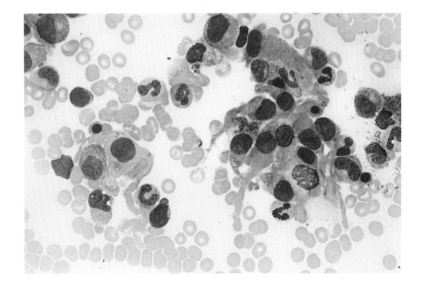

10.4. Langerhans cell histiocytosis
Bone marrow; α-mannosidase activity

The cells with long processes (see 10.3) exhibit intense focal α-mannosidase activity characteristic of Langerhans cell histiocytosis. Sometimes occasional rounded histiocytes, identical with those found in skin lesions, are present and these too show the intense focal α-mannosidase activity. Normal marrow cells have only weak diffuse activity at best. The abnormal cells would also be recognized using peanut agglutinin and CD1 antibodies.

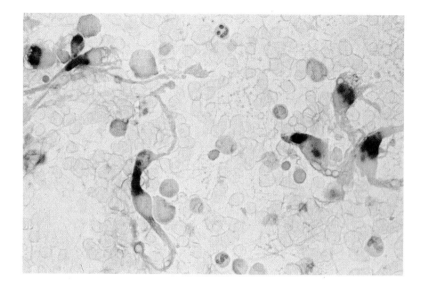

10.5. Langerhans cell histiocytosis
Bone marrow

Erythrophagocytosis, although rare in Langerhans cell histiocytosis, can occur.

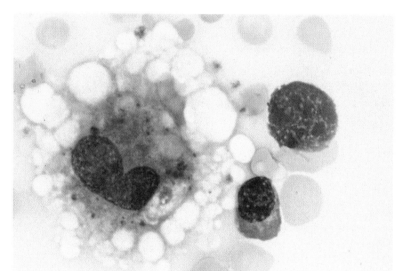

10.6. Langerhans cell histiocytosis
Bone marrow; iron stain

The presence of iron in macrophages indicates that a marked degree of erythrophagocytosis has taken place. However, erythrophagocytosis is a very non-specific phenomenon and occurs in a wide variety of situations ranging from Langerhans cell histiocytosis, familial erythrophagocytosis, and infection-associated haemophagocytic syndrome to post-transfusion states.

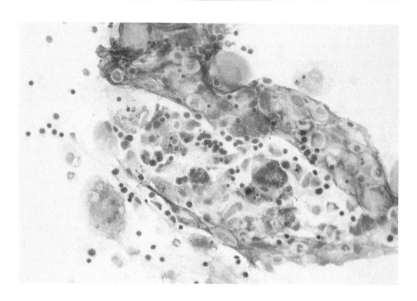

10.7. Langerhans cell histiocytosis
Electron photomicrograph
The striking appearance of the Birbeck granules (single arrows) identifies the probable Langerhans cell origin of the cell. Tennis racquet-like forms (double arrow) may also be seen and granules cut in cross section may be ring-like or target-like.

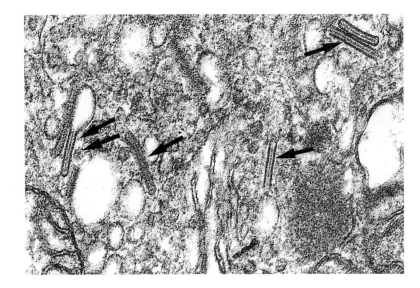

10.8. Langerhans cell histiocytosis
Lymph node; touch preparation
As shown here, the morphology of the histiocytes seen in this disorder can vary considerably and often includes mutlinucleate forms.

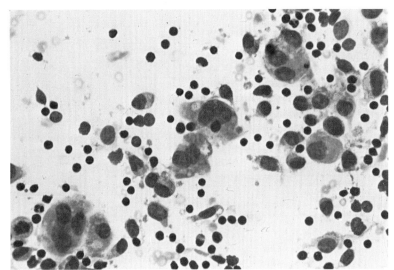

10.9. Familial erythrophagocytic lympho-histiocytosis
Lymph node; HE
This section shows many large macrophages full of ingested red cells. The patient presented (typically) at the age of six months, with pancytopenia, fever, lymphadenopathy and hepatosplenomegaly with jaundice. Lymph node biopsy, liver biopsy and bone marrow all revealed marked erythrophagocytosis. The patient had a sibling who had died with a similar disorder. The degree of erythrophagocytosis in the marrow may be minimal and the diagnosis on bone marrow aspirate is not usually possible.

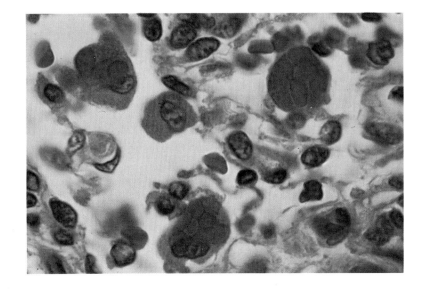

10.10. Familial erythrophagocytic lymphohistiocytosis
Lymph node; touch preparation

This shows two macrophages full of ingested red cells. The patient presented a similar clinical picture to that of the child whose biopsy is shown in 10.9. The diagnosis of familial erythrophagocytic lymphohistiocytosis is made by the combination of clinical features and family history, with the findings of high triglyceride levels and abnormal clotting factors. CNS involvement is frequent. Infection-associated haemophagocytic syndrome must be excluded.

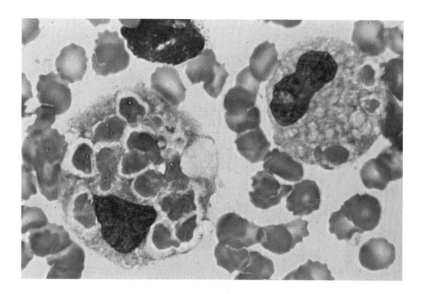

10.11. Infection-associated haemophagocytic syndrome
Bone marrow

This patient, aged 11 years, presented with recurrent fevers, bone pain, hepatosplenomegaly and pancytopenia. Erythrophagocytosis is present in this plate. The presence of haemophagocytosis is not a diagnostic feature, occurring in other situations (see 10.6), and isolation of a virus or other infective agent is a necessary part of the diagnosis.

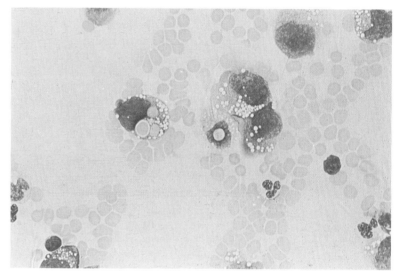

10.12. Infection-associated haemophagocytic syndrome
Bone marrow

Red cells, a normoblast, and a neutrophil have been ingested by a macrophage.

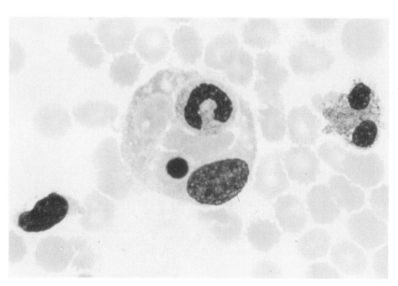

**10.13. Infection-associated
haemophagocytic syndrome**
Bone marrow
Platelets can also be ingested by
macrophages.

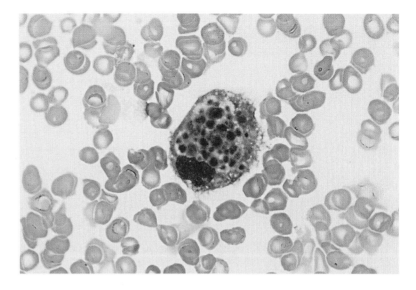

**10.14. Autoimmune disorder:
phagocytosis**
Bone marrow
In this composite picture histiocytes are
seen ingesting red cells, debris and nuclear
material. The sample was taken from a
12-year-old boy who was later diagnosed
as having dermatomyositis. The
haemophagocytosis was presumably
immune-mediated in this instance.

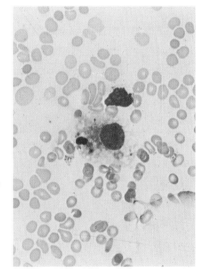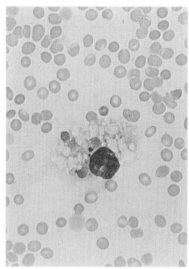

11
Lymphomas

Classification of childhood lymphomas (after updated Kiel)

1. Hodgkin's lymphoma

2. Non-Hodgkin's lymphoma
   (a) lymphoblastic lymphoma:
      (i)   B-lymphoblastic lymphoma, including Burkitt's lymphoma: arise in gut, Waldeyer's ring
      (ii) T-lymphoblastic lymphoma: present with mediastinal mass
     (iii) C-ALL lymphoblastic lymphoma: arise in bone, lymph nodes
   (b) peripheral T-cell lymphoma, including large cell anaplastic T-cell lymphoma (Ki-1 positive).

11.1. Normal lymph node
Touch preparation
The appearances of a normal lymph node are shown. The cut surface of the node is lightly pressed on to a glass slide and the imprint is fixed and stained. Lymphocytes are heterogeneous and scattered macrophages are seen.

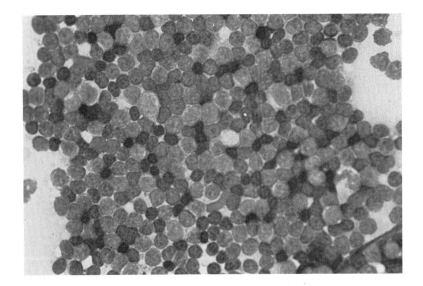

11.2. Non-Hodgkin's lymphoma
Lymph node; touch preparation
Compare with 11.1. There is a more homogeneous population of large blast cells, but normal appearances may vary especially in reactive nodes, and a confident diagnosis should not be made without histopathology and immunocytochemistry.

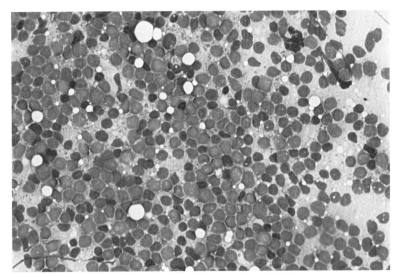

11.3. B-lymphoblastic lymphoma (Burkitt type)
Lymph node; touch preparation
This plate shows sheets of vacuolated blasts with interspersed macrophages. This so-called "starry sky" appearance is not specific and is seen in other lymphomas. The B-cell origin of this tumour was confirmed by immunocytochemistry.

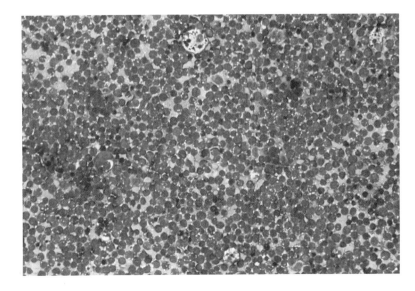

11.4. Normal lymph nodes
Touch preparation; acid
phosphatase

Some block positivity of T cells and strong
diffuse positivity of macrophages is shown.

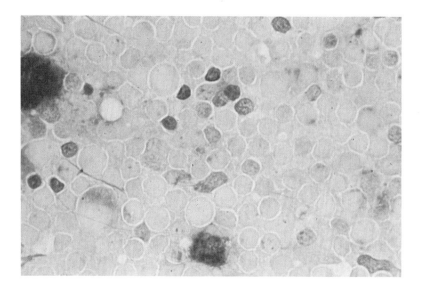

11.5. Non-Hodgkin's lymphoma
Touch preparation; acid
phosphatase

This preparation (same case as 11.2) shows
striking block positivity in most cells. A
T-lymphoblastic lymphoma was confirmed
by immunocytochemistry.

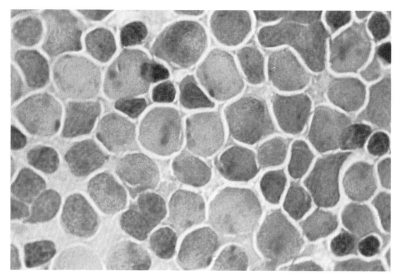

11.6. Hodgkin's lymphoma
Lymph node; touch preparation

A classical Reed–Sternberg cell with
double nuclei and 'owls eye' nucleoli is
shown.

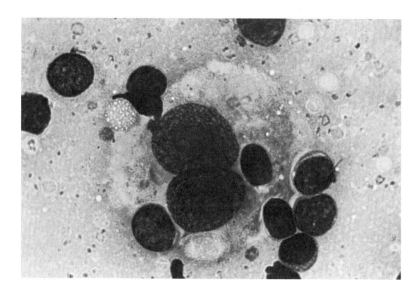

11.7. Hodgkin's lymphoma
Bone marrow trephine; HE
This eight-year-old girl presented with
fever and splenomegaly. There is a dense
fibrosis evident at low power. An increase
in reticulin may be the only evidence of
Hodgkin's lymphoma in bone marrow, and
along with an eosinophilia should make one
suspicious of this diagnosis in this clinical
setting.

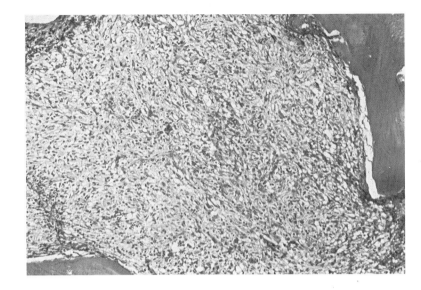

11.8. Hodgkin's lymphoma; pre-treatment
Bone marrow trephine; reticulin
This stain of the same sample shown in 11.7
clearly demonstrates the fibrosis commonly
present when Hodgkin's lymphoma
involves the marrow. Secondary
myelofibrosis may also be present without
overt tumour invasion.

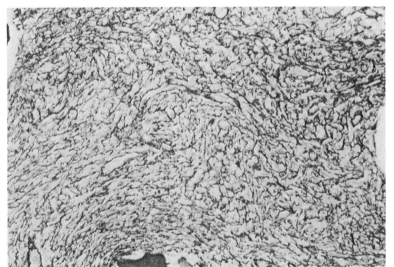

11.9. Hodgkin's lymphoma; after chemotherapy
Bone marrow trephine; reticulin
Just after the trephine biopsy, shown in
11.8 was taken, the patient was treated
with quadruple chemotherapy. Six months
later she was in complete remission and the
bone marrow trephine showed no evidence
of fibrosis.

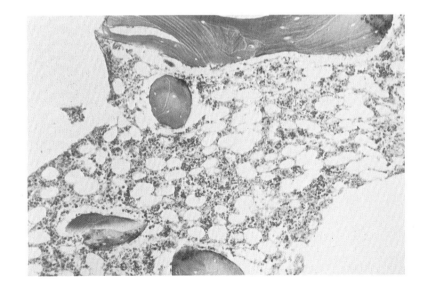

12
Other tumours

12.1. Small round cell tumour of childhood
Touch preparation; marrow trephine

Clumps of tumour cells are seen with free tumour cells in the surrounding areas. Accurate diagnosis of small round cell tumours is difficult in bone marrow aspirates. Plastic sections of trephines to give better morphology will help but tissue diagnosis on the primary tumour is essential.

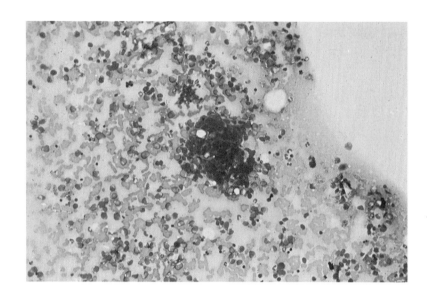

12.2. Small round cell tumour of childhood
Touch preparation; marrow trephine

Clumps of tumour cells are seen which on high-power examination show vacuolation. Differentiation of solid tumours is impossible in this type of preparation.

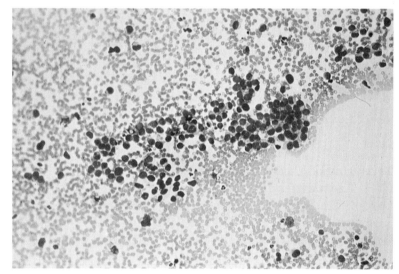

12.3. Neuroblastoma
Bone marrow
This plate shows a clump of tumour cells in an otherwise normal marrow.

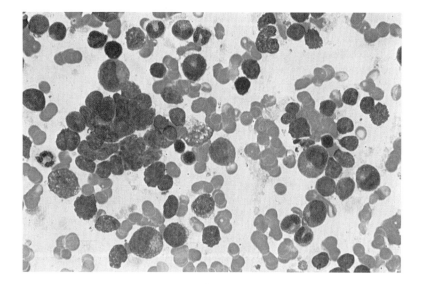

12.4. Neuroblastoma
Bone marrow
This sample was taken from the right iliac crest of a patient whose left iliac crest sample showed only rare tumour cells. This marrow is almost replaced by malignant cells which are forming sheets rather than rosettes. Marrow infiltration by neuroblastoma may be patchy.

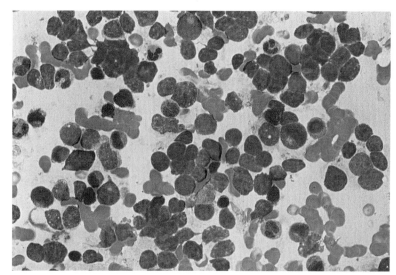

12.5. Neuroblastoma
Bone marrow
High-power view of a clump of tumour cells. The cells can usually be distinguished from lymphoma/leukaemia cells by their patchy distribution, their tendency to clump and by the relatively low nuclear:cytoplasmic ratio.

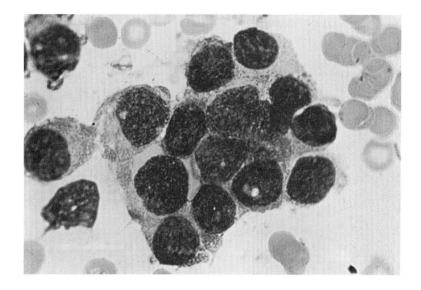

12.6. Neuroblastoma
   Bone marrow
This shows complete replacement of
marrow by tumour cells which are
vacuolated. This degree of vacuolation is,
however, unusual. The patient, aged 18
months, had a large adrenal mass. The
clinical picture, with cell surface marker
studies (see 12.7), and a raised urinary
VMA gave the diagnosis, which was
confirmed on the resected tumour.
Vacuolation may also be seen in
rhabdomyosarcoma (12.17) and Ewing's
tumour (12.12).

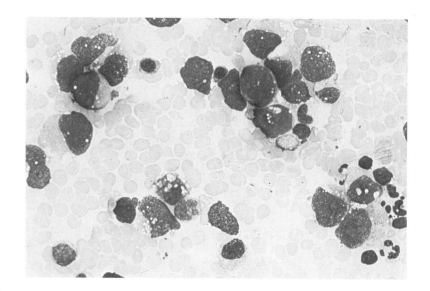

12.7. Neuroblastoma
   Bone marrow
A group of cells is detected by fluorescein-
labelled antibody UJ 13A (left) among a
bigger cluster of cells seen by phase-
contrast microscopy (right). Care is needed
in the interpretation of preparations stained
with this antibody as it is known to cross-
react with osteoblasts. (Oppedal and
Kemshead, personal communication).

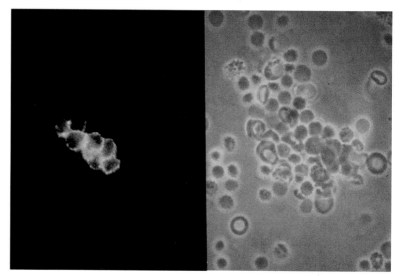

12.8. Neuroblastoma
   Bone marrow trephine; plastic
   section
Thin sections of resin-embedded trephines
offer much better morphology and
cytological detail than paraffin sections.
Neuroblastoma cells with prominent
nucleoli are readily identified in this plate.

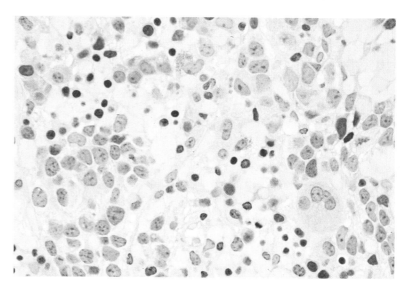

12.9. Neuroblastoma
Pleural fluid; cytocentrifuge

This cytospin deposit from a pleural effusion contains tumour cells (a) surrounded by lymphocytes (b), and macrophages (c). See accompanying diagram for the identification of the cells. It may be difficult to distinguish normal reactive mesothelial cells and malignant cells in an effusion.

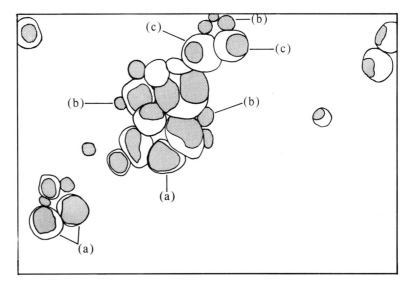

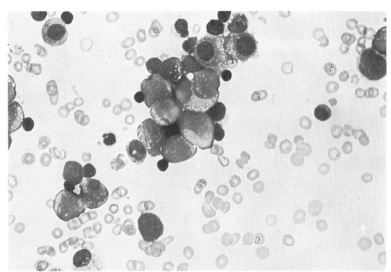

12.10. Neuroblastoma
Lymph node; touch preparation

Here a clump of tumour cells is seen. Touch preparations are useful for rapid diagnosis of tumour in involved lymph nodes but histological studies are invariably required for the precise diagnosis of a solid tumour.

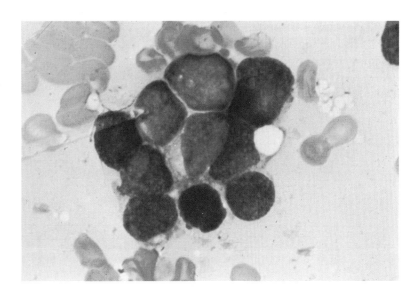

12.11. Ewing's tumour
Bone marrow

A primary, osteolytic tumour was present in the pelvis. The marrow is replaced by a heterogeneous population of vacuolated tumour cells. There are no specific features and other tumours such as L3-type ALL, non-Hodgkin's lymphoma, neuroblastoma and rhabdomyosarcoma must be considered. The PAS stain is often positive (12.13), but this reaction may also be present in rhabdomyosarcoma and lymphoblastic leukaemia.

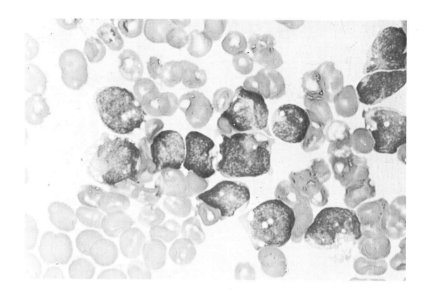

12.12. Ewing's tumour
Bone marrow

High-power view of a tumour cell showing vacuolation, which also occurs in other situations (see 12.11).

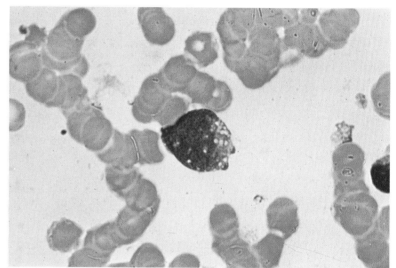

12.13. Ewing's tumour
Bone marrow; PAS

The tumour cells contain glycogen and are PAS-positive. A PAS-positive normal neutrophil is also present.

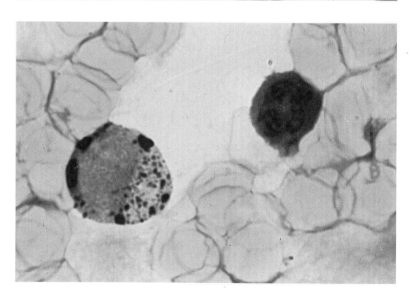

12.14. Ewing's tumour
Bone marrow trephine; HE
Vacuolation of the cytoplasm of the tumour cells is evident, and appears as empty blebs in some cells.

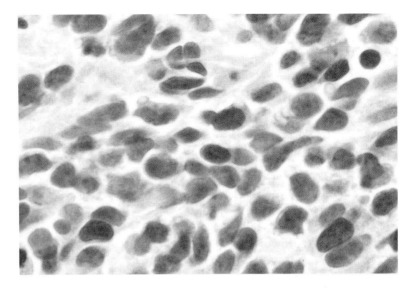

12.15. Ewing's tumour
Bone marrow trephine; PAS
The vacuoles and blebs are PAS-positive.

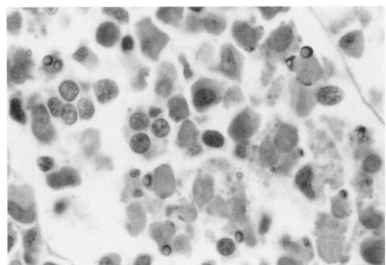

12.16. Askin tumour (primitive neuroectodermal tumour)
Pleural fluid
Spun deposit from a 12-year-old girl with a massive pleural effusion. A clump of cells is seen. The original diagnosis on tissue excised at thoracotomy was Ewing's tumour but recent review and marker studies indicated an Askin tumour.

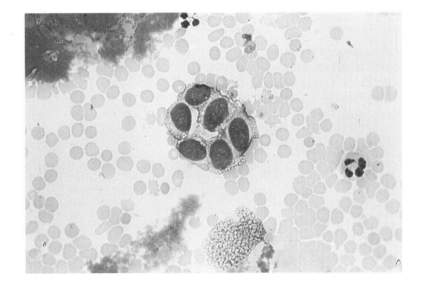

12.17. Rhabdomyosarcoma
Touch preparation; marrow trephine

A clump of tumour cells with cytoplasmic vacuolation is seen. Accurate diagnosis is not possible without further investigation as similar vacuolation may be seen in neuroblastoma, and in lymphoblastic leukaemia and Burkitt's lymphoma.

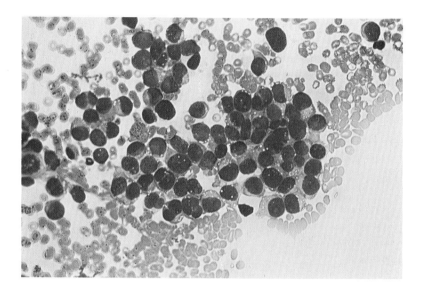

12.18. Rhabdomyosarcoma
Bone marrow

In this case the tumour cells show marked vacuolation.

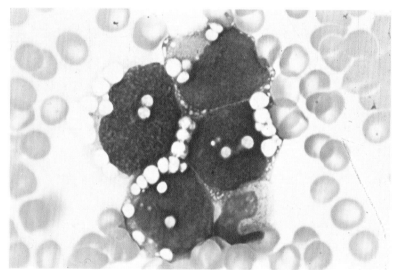

12.19. Rhabdomyosarcoma
Bone marrow; PAS

The tumour cells contain masses of PAS-positive blocks. A similar pattern may be seen in Ewing's tumour (12.13) and in lymphoblastic (L1 and L2) leukaemia.

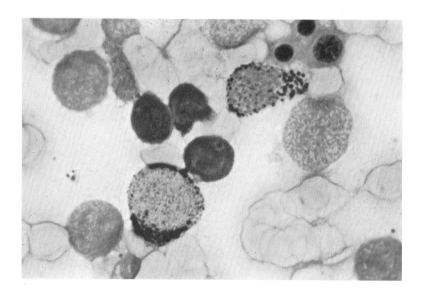

12.20. Rhabdomyosarcoma
Bone marrow trephine; HE
The tumour cells have pale nuclei and are spindle shaped but are effectively camouflaged within normal haematopoietic tissue on low-power viewing.

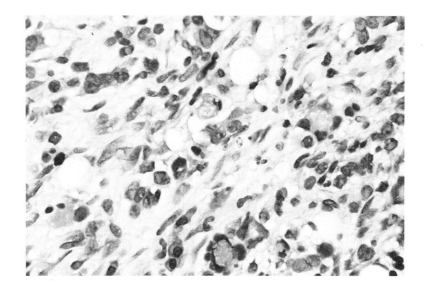

12.21. Rhabdomyosarcoma
Bone marrow trephine; immunocytochemical demonstration of desmin
The presence of desmin (yellow-brown) within the tumour cells indicates a myogenic origin and confirms the diagnosis of rhabdomyosarcoma. Other small round cell tumours are desmin negative.

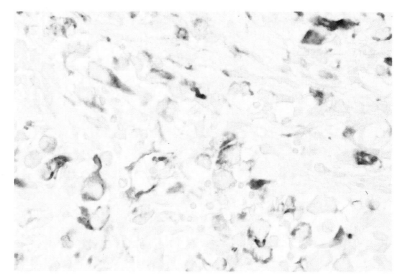

12.22. Malignant germ-cell tumour: seminoma with yolk sac elements
Bone marrow trephine
A 12-year-old boy presented with leucoerythroblastic anaemia, bone pain and a mediastinal mass. In this marrow trephine there is near complete replacement of normal haemopoiesis by malignant cells—an almost unprecedented occurrence in malignant germ-cell tumours.

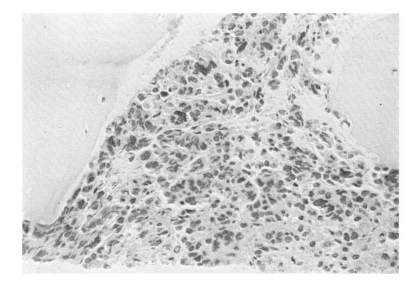

12.23. Malignant germ-cell tumour: seminoma with yolk sac elements

Mediastinal mass; stained to show alphafetoprotein

Yolk sac (endodermal sinus) differentiation is demonstrated by the presence of AFP (yellow-brown) in the cells on the right of the picture. Same case as 12.22.

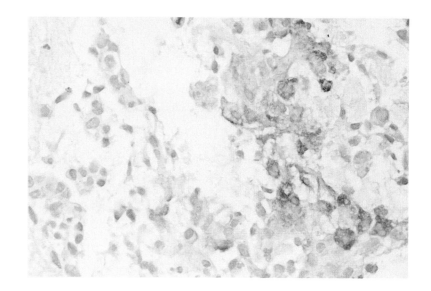

12.24. Ependymoma

Bone marrow aspirate

Clumps of tumour cells are seen. They have no specific identifying features. This is a rare instance of metastatic ependymoma in a seven-year-old boy who, two years before, had a ventriculo-atrial shunt inserted at the time of partial removal of a posterior cranial fossa tumour.

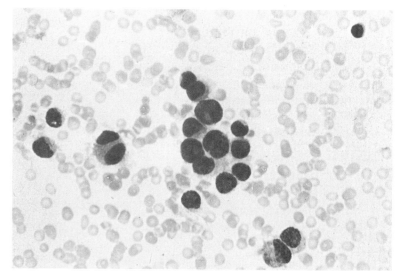

12.25. Ependymoma

Bone marrow trephine; HE

Trephine biopsy from the same patient as in 12.24 showing areas of tumour infiltration and reactive fibrosis alongside some normal haemopoiesis.

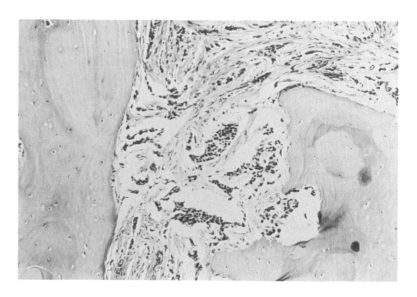

12.26. Medulloblastoma

Bone marrow trephine; HE
There is infiltration by tumour cells with some normal marrow activity. In other areas there was extension of tumour into vascular spaces and marked reactive fibrosis. The bone felt abnormally hard on biopsy and no aspirate was obtained. The incidence of extracranial metastasis may be higher in the patient with a ventriculosystemic shunt, but this 14-year-old girl had no such shunt.

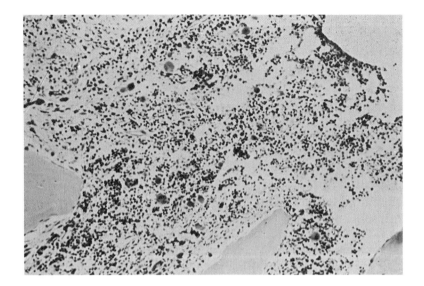

13
Aplastic anaemia

13.1. Fanconi's anaemia
Bone marrow trephine biopsy;
HE

This disorder is a constitutional aplastic
anaemia: constitutional disorders
associated with marrow hypoplasia include
dyskeratosis congenita and familial aplasia
without congenital anomalies (Estren and
Dameshek).

In Fanconi's anaemia the congenital
anomalies are usually noted by early
infancy but haematological changes are
rarely evident before 18 months and can
be delayed until the second decade.
Thrombocytopenia often precedes the
development of pancytopenia. In this 12-
year-old boy, marrow hypoplasia had
become severe. As with other conditions
displaying chromosome breakages, there is
a strong association with development of
leukaemia. This child died of acute myeloid
leukaemia. See 2.62 and 2.63 for
dyserythropoietic changes in this disorder.

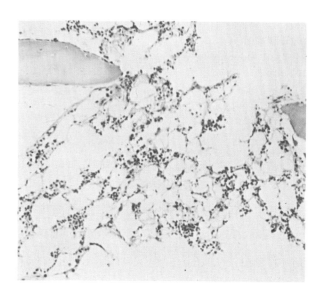

13.2. Idiopathic acquired aplastic anaemia
Bone marrow trephine biopsy;
HE

Most cases of aplastic anaemia in childhood
are acquired and no cause is found. The
marrow biopsy shows the patchy but
markedly reduced cellularity and increased
fat spaces typical of this disorder.

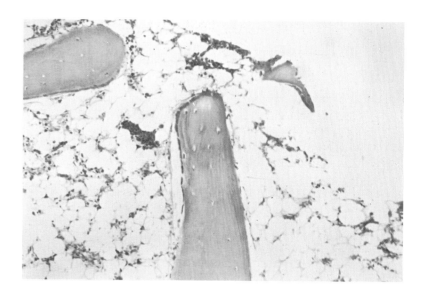

13.3. Aplastic anaemia
Blood film; Kleihauer stain
(ref. 5)

Hb F-containing red cells are demonstrated because of their resistance to acid elution. In some patients with aplastic anaemia the Hb F is raised, occasionally as high as 15 per cent. This plate shows an increased percentage of cells in a heterogeneous distribution. Some 'ghost' cells contain little or no Hb F.

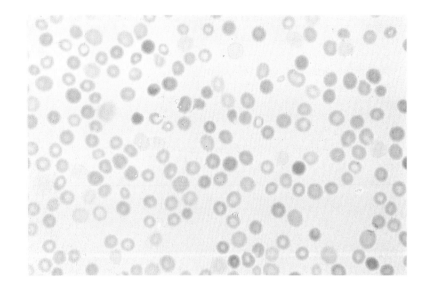

13.4. Post-hepatitis marrow aplasia
Bone marrow

Aplastic anaemia following hepatitis A carries a poor prognosis. A bone marrow particle with greatly decreased cellularity is shown.

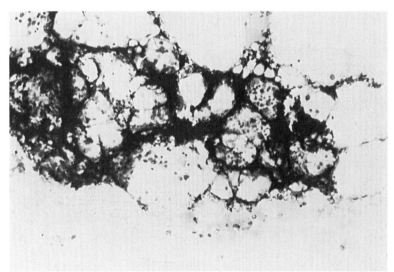

13.5. Post-cytotoxic chemotherapy aplasia
Bone marrow trephine biopsy;
HE

The cellularity is grossly decreased following a course of intensive chemotherapy in a patient with RAEB. Similar appearances may be seen following ablative chemo-radiotherapy as conditioning for bone marrow transplantation.

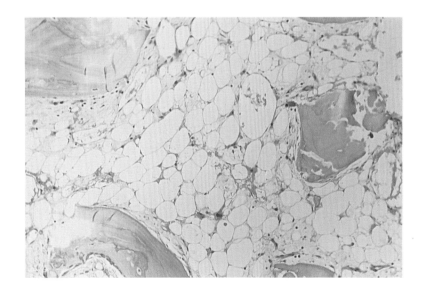

13.6. Hereditary spherocytosis—parvovirus-induced aplasia
Blood film

A seven-year-old boy with hereditary spherocytosis presented with an 'aplastic crisis' (Hb 4.5 g/dl and reticulocytopenia). IgM to parvovirus B19 was demonstrated.

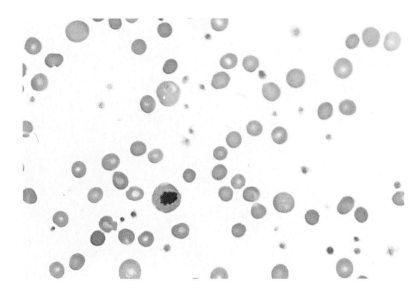

13.7 and 13.8. Parvovirus-induced aplasia
Bone marrow

Parvovirus can cause aplasia of other marrow elements although it usually produces severe anaemia. It has recently been recognized that bizarre giant cells are often present in the marrow in these cases. Sometimes these present as bare nuclei and others resemble early pronormoblasts. They always have very prominent nucleoli.

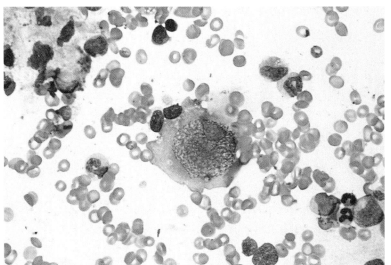

13.8. Parvovirus-induced aplasia
Bone marrow; see 13.7

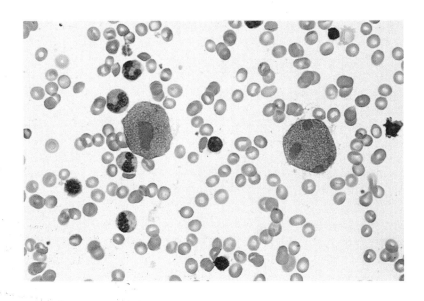

14
Neonatal and perinatal disorders

14.1. Fetal blood
Blood film

This blood sample was taken via a fetoscope from a mother with thalassaemia minor, to exclude homozygous beta thalassaemia in the child. There is relative macrocytosis (MCV 100 fl). A single nucleated red cell is seen.

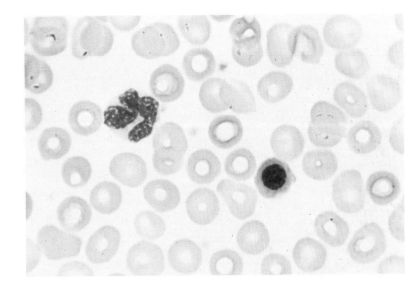

14.2. Cord blood
Blood film

Sample from a healthy normal-term baby. There is anisocytosis with macrocytes and a few circulating nucleated red cells. Irregularly contracted cells are also common.

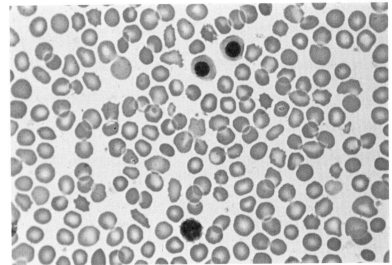

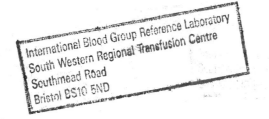

14.3. Neonatal marrow
Bone marrow
There are fewer erythroblasts and more lymphocytes in neonatal marrows compared with those of older children.

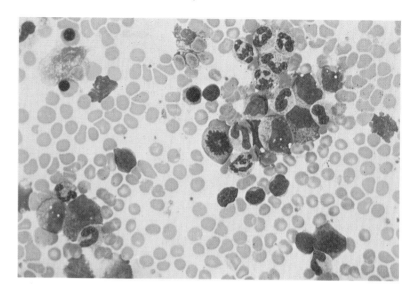

14.4. The 'stressed' neonate— respiratory distress syndrome (RDS)
Blood film
Poikilocytosis and irregularly contracted cells are common features of blood films from sick neonates, sometimes giving rise to the nebulous diagnosis of 'infantile pyknocytosis', an ill-defined entity best ignored. Premature infant of 27 weeks on day 3.

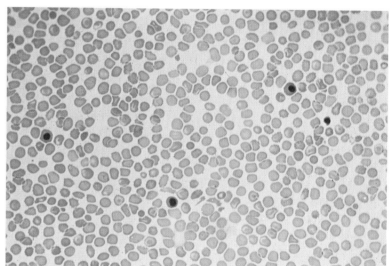

14.5. The 'stressed' neonate— respiratory distress syndrome
Blood film
Twenty-four week premature baby, two days postnatal. Haemoglobin 11.1 g/dl.

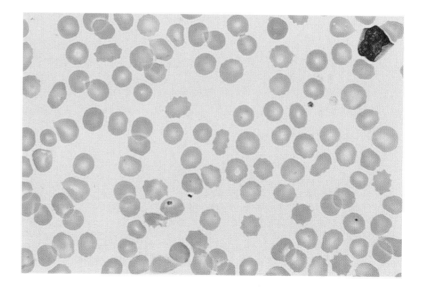

**14.6. The 'stressed' neonate—
respiratory distress syndrome**
Blood film
Nucleated red cells and Howell—Jolly
bodies indicate functional hyposplenism.
Same patient as 14.4.

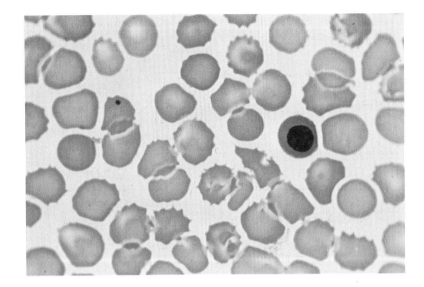

**14.7. The 'stressed' neonate—
respiratory distress syndrome**
Blood film
RDS is an occasional cause of consumption
coagulopathy (disseminated intravascular
coagulation) as in this case where marked
red cell changes are associated with
profound thrombocytopenia.

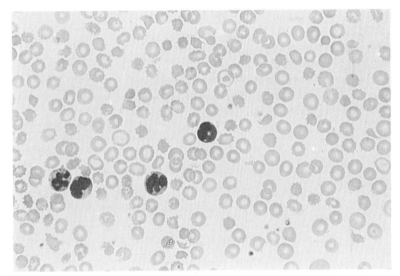

14.8. The 'stressed' neonate—sepsis
Blood film
One-day-old term neonate with a
septicaemia. Note spherocytes and band-
form neutrophil.

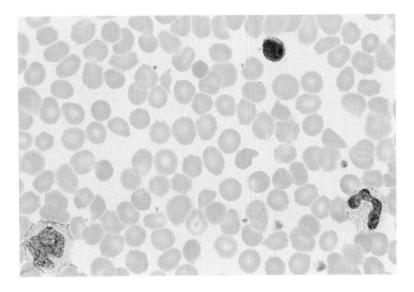

14.9. The 'stressed' neonate—sepsis
Blood film

Immature granulocytes in another neonatal septicaemia.

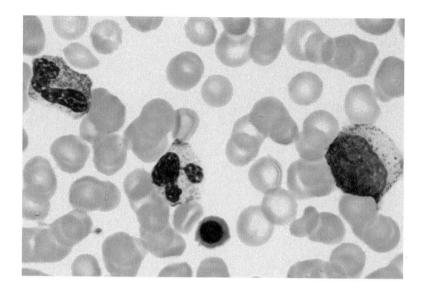

14.10. The 'stressed' neonate—sepsis
Blood film

Disseminated intravascular coagulation commonly complicates neonatal septicaemia. In this example gross red cell changes are associated with profound thrombocytopenia.

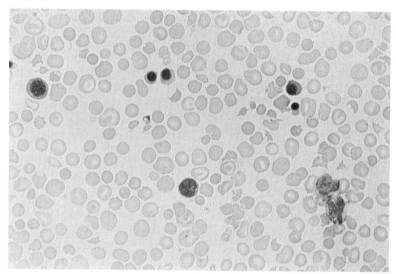

14.11. The 'stressed' neonate—sepsis
Blood film

Twelve-day-old neonate with a tracheo-oesophageal fistula and pneumonia. Pyknocytosis, polychromasia and anisocytosis.

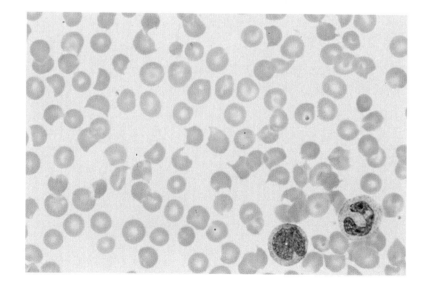

14.12. The 'stressed' neonate— meconium ileus
Blood film
A one-day-old term baby with cystic fibrosis and meconium ileus. Absolute nucleated red cell count $16 \times 10^9/l$.

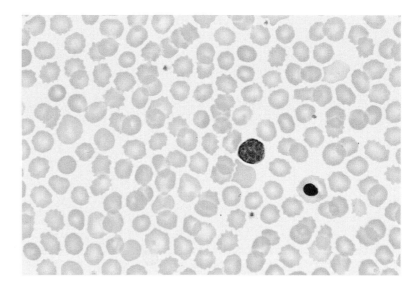

14.13. The 'stressed' neonate— congenital heart disease
Blood film
Similar red cell abnormalities can be produced by a variety of different pathological conditions in the neonatal period.

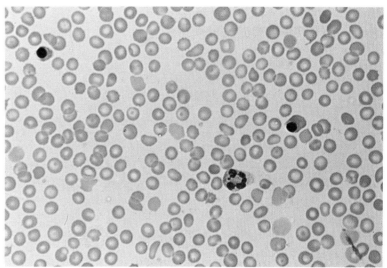

14.14. Haemolytic disease of the newborn—feto:maternal haemorrhage
Kleihauer film of maternal blood
Shows a massive transplacental haemorrhage with 20 000 fetal cells per 50 low-power fields.

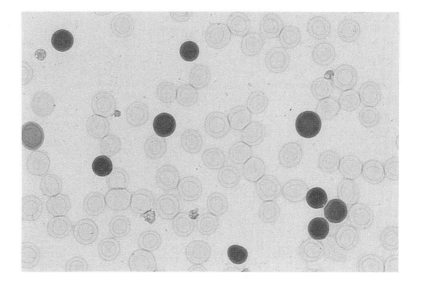

14.15. Haemolytic disease of the newborn—feto:maternal haemorrhage
Blood film (maternal)
Shows macrocyte of probable fetal origin. The baby was born anaemic (7 g/dl) with no evidence of haemolysis.

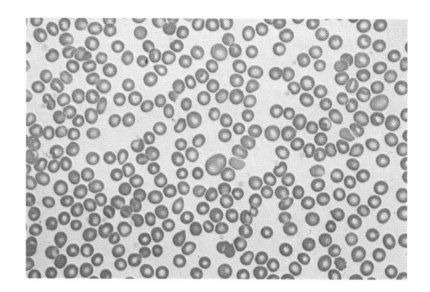

14.16. Haemolytic disease of the newborn—isoimmune due to anti-D
Blood film (cord blood)
Numerous erythroblasts and polychromatic macrocytes; occasional spherocytes; anaemia.

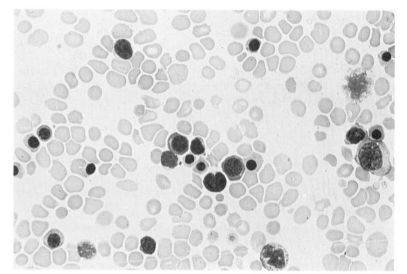

14.17. Haemolytic disease of the newborn—ABO haemolytic disease
Blood film
Usually less severe than Rhesus haemolytic disease, with a negative or only weakly positive direct AHG test, ABO disease presents 24–72 h after birth. Spherocytes are a feature rather than an occasional finding.

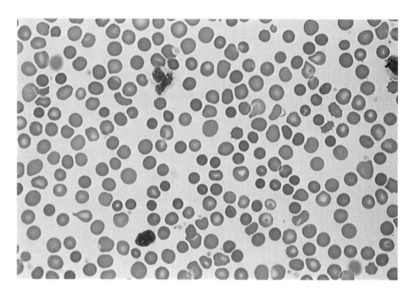

14.18. Haemolytic disease of the newborn—ABO haemolytic disease
Blood film
A severe example presenting 12 h after birth. Haemoglobin 14.1 g/dl. Bilirubin at 24 h, 470 μmol/l; reticulocytes 730 × 10^9/l.

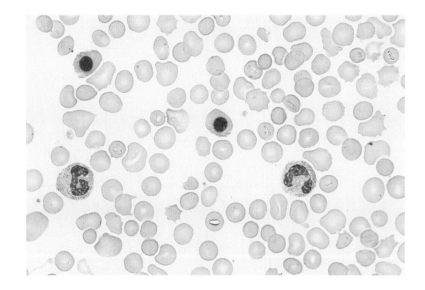

14.19. 'TORCH' infection—cytomegalovirus
Bone marrow
All the congenital 'TORCH' infections (toxoplasmosis, rubella, cytomegalovirus and herpes simplex) together with congenital syphilis can produce a similar haematological picture in the neonate, with hepatosplenomegaly, jaundice, anaemia and thrombocytopenia. The marrow (as in this case) may contain cells morphologically similar to lymphoblasts. The baby was born with purpura and hepatosplenomegaly. Confusion with congenital leukaemia can arise.

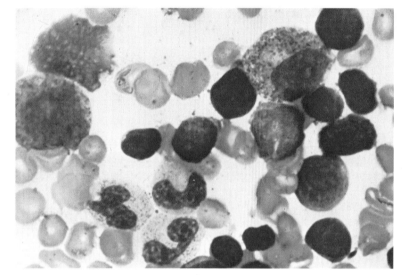

14.20 and 14.21. 'TORCH' infection—cytomegalovirus
Bone marrow
Further material from the same patient as 14.19.

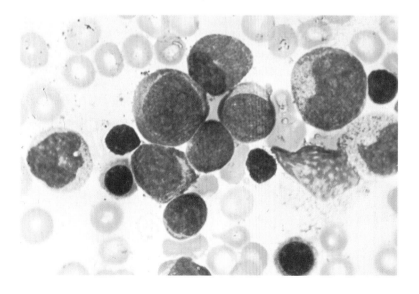

14.21. Cytomegalovirus
Bone marrow
Same patient as 14.19.

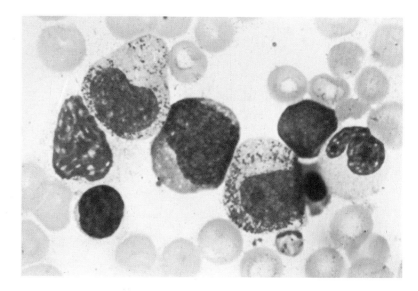

14.22. Reticular dysgenesis
Bone marrow
This child suffered recurrent infections
starting in the neonatal period. At the age
of nine months he was shown to have
neutropenia, lymphopenia, and absent
serum immunoglobulins. Reticular
dysgenesis, a very rare form of severe
combined immune deficiency, was
diagnosed. The bone marrow shows
depletion of lymphoid and granulocyte
precursors, particularly mature forms. The
baby was successfully treated by allogeneic
bone marrow transplantation.

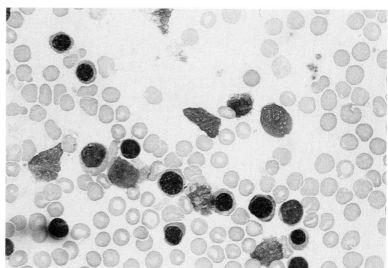

14.23. Infantile osteopetrosis
Blood film
Gross leucoerythroblastosis can
occasionally be confused with leukaemia.
The patient was a six-month-old boy
presenting with pallor (Hb 8.7 g/dl) and
massive splenomegaly. The condition is an
inherited functional deficiency of
osteoclasts.

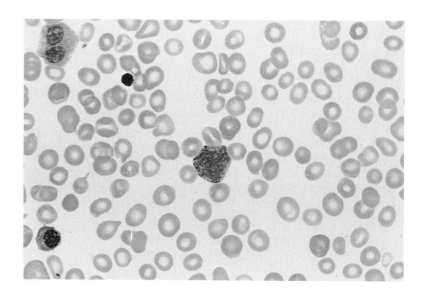

14.24. Infantile osteopetrosis
Bone marrow trephine
Dense cancellous bone with constricted
marrow space.

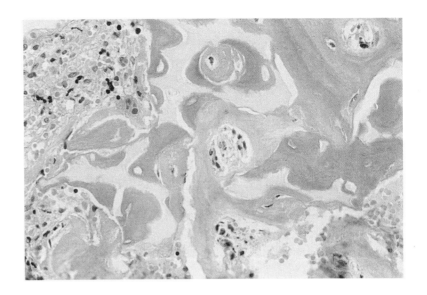

15
Parasites and opportunistic infections

15.1. Malaria; *Plasmodium vivax,*
early trophozoites (signet forms)
Blood film

This plate shows two cells infected with trophozoites. One of them contains three distinct signet forms—a single parasite is much more usual. There are no 'Schuffner's dots' (see 15.2) present.

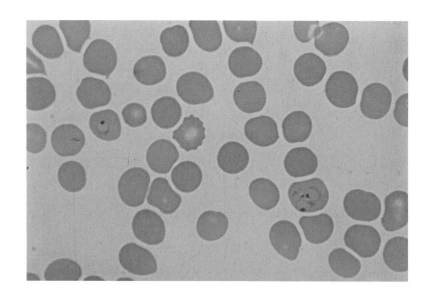

15.2. Malaria: *Plasmodium vivax,*
developing trophozoite
Blood film

The red cell at the centre contains a single trophozoite and also numerous Schuffner's dots. These dots, staining pink with MGG or Leishman's stain, are helpful in distinguishing *P. vivax* from other forms of malaria, but should not be confused with intra-parasite pigment granules.

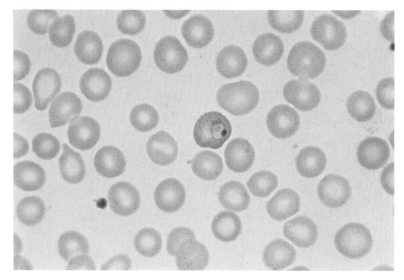

15.3. Malaria; *Plasmodium vivax,*
   developing trophozoites
   Blood film
The parasite shows a coarse irregular
shape, chromatin, which appears as dots or
threads, and scattered fine yellow-brown
pigment.

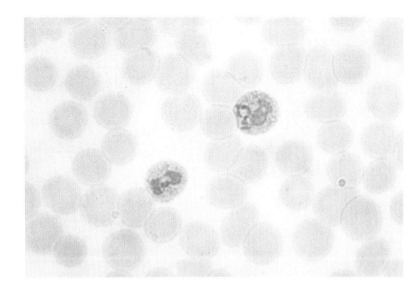

15.4. Malaria; *Plasmodium vivax,*
   schizonts
   Blood film
The non-segmented schizonts represent a
phase of the asexual cycle later than the
trophozoite.

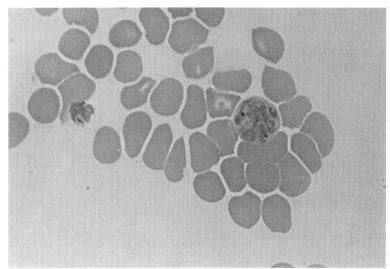

15.5. Malaria; *Plasmodium vivax,*
   schizonts
   Blood film
Gradual concentration of chromatin occurs
prior to the final development of
merozoites.

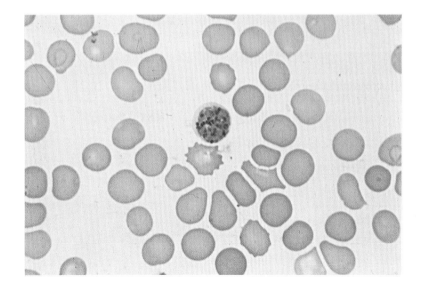

15.6. Malaria; *Plasmodium vivax,*
   schizogony
   Blood film
The plate shows a segmented schizont just
prior to separation of individual
merozoites.

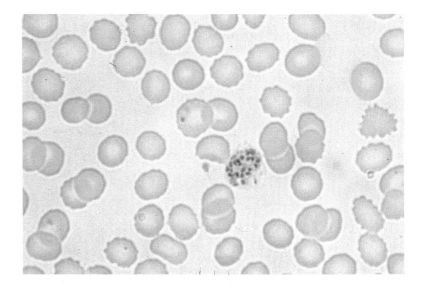

15.7. Malaria; *Plasmodium vivax,*
   microgametocytes
   Blood film
The microgametocytes may be numerous in
the blood film. They fill the enlarged red
cell and contain numerous pigment
granules.

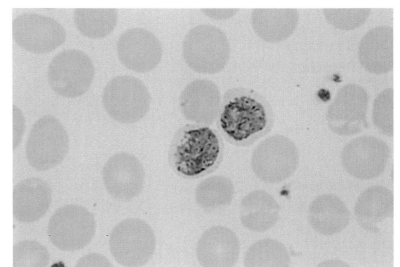

15.8. Malaria; *Plasmodium vivax*
   Bone marrow film
Occasional ring trophozoite forms were
found in the bone marrow from this patient
who presented with hepatosplenomegaly
and fever. No parasites were initially
detected in the peripheral blood.

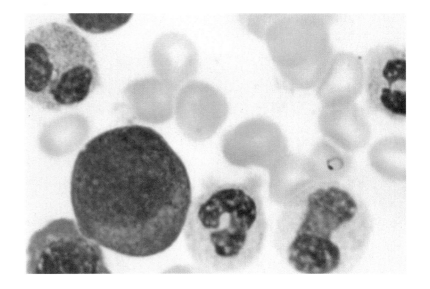

15.9. Malaria; *Plasmodium falciparum*, **ring trophozoite**
'Thin' blood film

The ring form of the trophozoite of *P. falciparum* is smaller and more delicate than that of *P. vivax*. Multiple-infected cells are common. Maurer's clefts (finer than Schuffner's dots) are common in the developing trophozoite but not seen in this particular preparation; their origin is unknown.

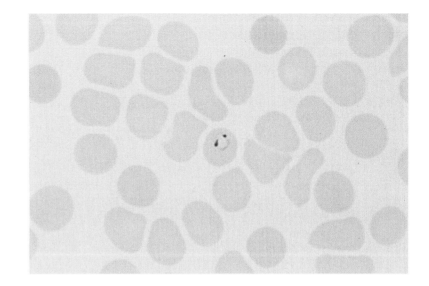

15.10. Malaria; *Plasmodium falciparum*
Blood film

Segmented mature schizonts containing six to twelve merozoites are present in this illustration (lower right) together with a signet form of trophozoite (upper left).

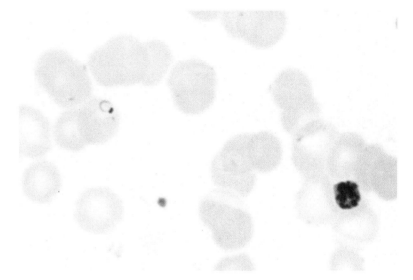

15.11. Malaria; *Plasmodium falciparum*
'Thick' blood film

The thick film, in skilled hands, is quick to make and is the best preparation for general clinical use. The technique is well described in standard texts (see references). By this method, all red cells are lysed and the diagnostic chromatin dots consequently stand out. This particular plate shows a *P. falciparum* infection but all other types of malaria may be diagnosed by the method. The heavily stained cells are white blood cells.

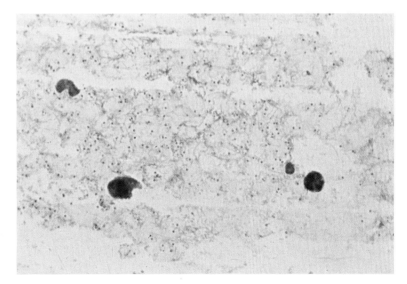

15.12. Malaria; *Plasmodium falciparum* **(sexual cycle)** Blood film
The male gametocyte ('microgametocyte') is shown in this plate. The pink and blue cytoplasm is characteristic and pigment is distributed throughout the large nucleus.

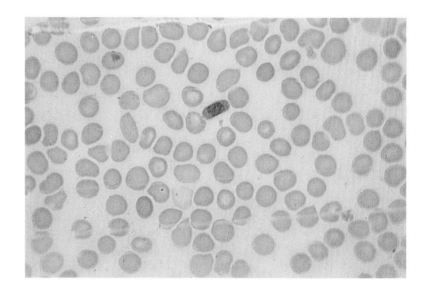

15.13. Malaria; *Plasmodium falciparum* **(sexual cycle)** Blood film
The female gametocyte ('macrogametocyte'), with its sharply rounded or pointed ends and its dense, small nucleus, is illustrated here. The cytoplasm is typically deeper blue than that of the male gametocyte.

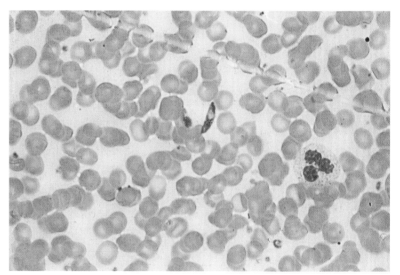

15.14. Malaria; *Plasmodium ovale* Blood film
Developing trophozoite: this occupies up to one-third of the red cell, which becomes irregular and pointed. Schuffner's dots are present.

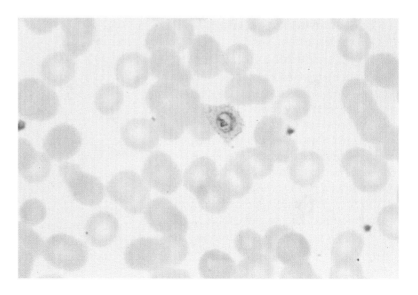

15.15. Malaria; *Plasmodium*
 malariae
 Blood film
Schizonts are very similar to those of *P. ovale*.

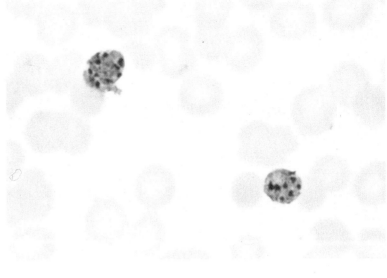

15.16. Malaria; *Plasmodium*
 malariae
 Blood film
Macrogametocyte, very similar to *P. vivax*.

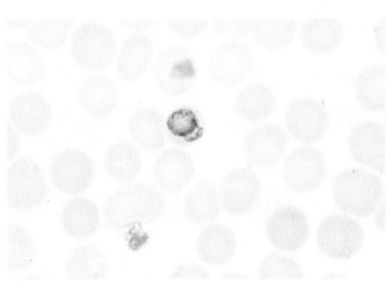

15.17. Leishmaniasis (kala-azar)
 Bone marrow aspirate
The three-year-old patient had just returned, with fever and hepatosplenomegaly, to the UK after a holiday in Jordan. Each parasite (Leishman–Donovan body) has a dense trophonucleus and a less densely staining kinetoplast.

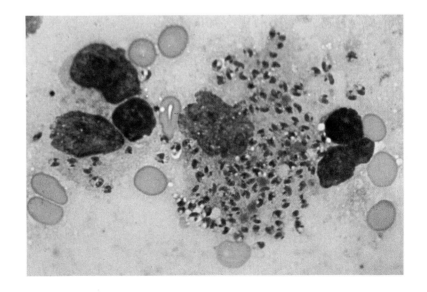

15.18. Leishmaniasis (kala-azar)
Bone marrow trephine
The parasites are readily visible in
histological sections stained by HE.

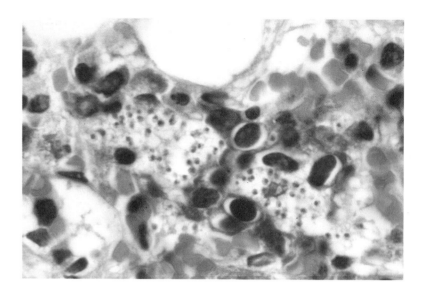

15.19. *Trypanosoma rhodesiense*
(Rhodesian sleeping sickness)
Blood film
These parasites are transmitted by the
tsetse fly. This patient had been on a
hunting expedition to the Zambezi Valley
and presented with an encephalitic illness.
The plate shows the parasite's undulating
membrane, flagellum, nucleus, and
kinetoplast.

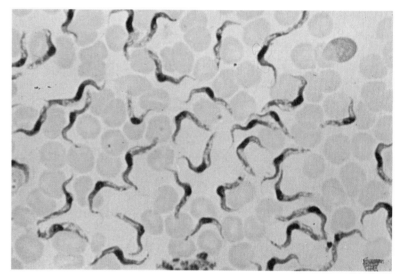

15.20. *Trypanosoma rhodesiense*
(Rhodesian sleeping sickness)
Blood film
The undulating membrane, central
nucleus and kinetoplast are shown. The
appearances are indistinguishable from *T.
gambiense*, but the chronic nature of *T.
gambiense* infection helps to differentiate it
from the more acute effect of *T.
rhodesiense*.

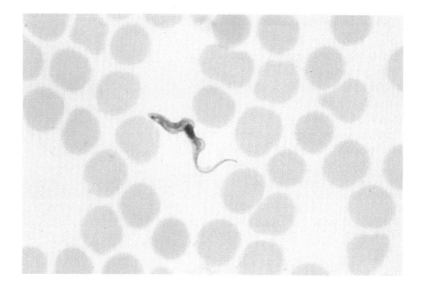

15.21. *Trypanosoma cruzi* (Chagas' disease)
Blood film

This parasite is indigenous to South America. It has a very large terminal kinetoplast, a large nucleus, and is typically 'C-shaped'. Clinical presentation in children is usually with remitting fever, lymphadenopathy, oedema, and lesions of skin ('chagomas') or conjunctiva (Romana's sign). Myocarditis, encephalitis and intestinal dysfunction also occur. *T. cruzi* metamorphose in tissue macrophages and have leishmanial forms.

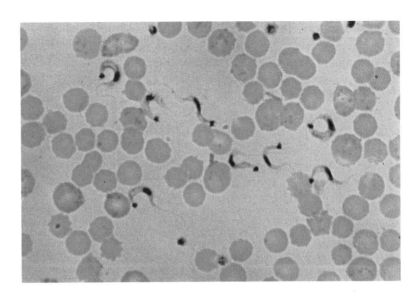

15.22. Microfilariasis; *Wuchereria bancrofti*
Blood film

Filariae are members of the Nematoda. Their larval forms—microfilariae—are found in the blood, especially at night, as demonstrated here. Chronic consequences of filarial infection include lymphangitis and elephantiasis, though the latter is very rare in childhood. *Wuchereria bancrofti* is sheathed and the nuclei do not extend to the tip of the tail. *Brugia malayi* is similar in its habit and form; the nuclei extend to the tail and the larvae are sheathed. Microfilariae of other species may be found in blood (e.g., *Dipetalonema perstans*, *Dipetalonema streptocerca* and *Mansonella ozzardi*). These are unsheathed and seem to be nonpathogenic.

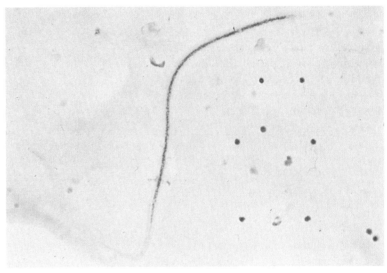

15.23. Loa-loa ('Calabar swelling')
Blood film

These microfilariae are transmitted by flies of the Chrysops genus and will develop into adult worms that cause soft-tissue swellings, especially on the hands, arms, and eyelids. Although the infection may be chronic, the prognosis for life is excellent. These microfilariae, unlike those of *W. bancrofti* (see 15.22) are most easily demonstrated in a daytime blood film.

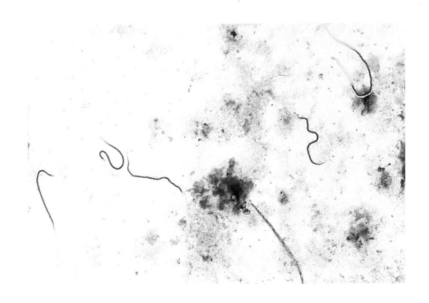

15.24. Loa-loa
Blood film

The microfilariae are sheathed and measure up to 300 μm long. Nuclei extend to the tip of the tail.

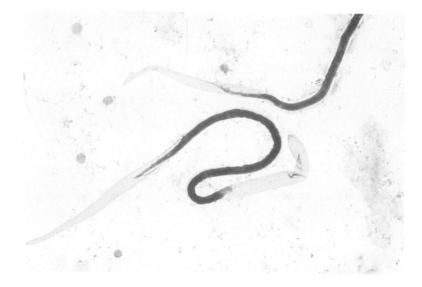

15.25. Babesia
Blood film

Babesiosis is a tick-borne disease, with mild symptoms of fever, malaise and haemolytic anaemia. The organisms are present in red cells and have a variety of appearances. Here the coccoid form is seen.

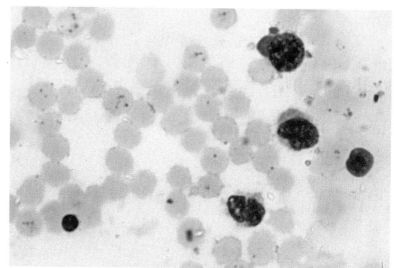

15.26. Babesia
Blood film

The organism also has some resemblance to the ring trophozoite form of *Plasmodium falciparum*.

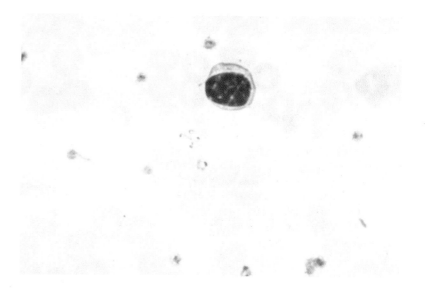

15.27. Borrelia
Blood film

Lyme disease is caused by the tick-borne spirochaete *Borrelia recurrentis* and gives rise to relapsing fevers and joint pains.

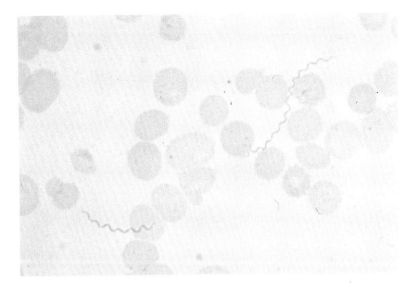

15.28. *Candida albicans* (Moniliasis)
Bone marrow trephine; HE

This teenage patient had had a bone marrow transplant for leukaemia 3 months before. Haemopoietic reconstitution had occurred but the patient developed persistent fever. *C. albicans* was cultured from both blood and bone marrow; the fungus (mostly hyphal forms) is readily detected in this trephine biopsy.

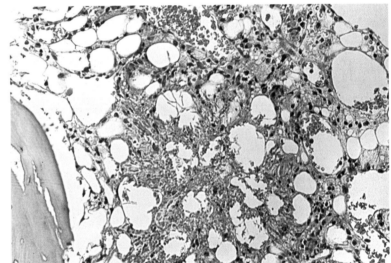

16
Storage disorders

NIEMANN–PICK DISEASE

16.1. Niemann–Pick disease (type A, infantile)
Bone marrow

Foamy cells, generally with uniform sized vacuoles in any one cell, are prominent throughout the film. Rarely nuclear debris or an occasional engulfed erythrocyte may be present. Vacuolated lymphocytes may be found in the blood. Patients with this disorder present in early infancy with hepatosplenomegaly and failure to thrive. Mental retardation is usually apparent but may not occur until one year of age. Sphingomyelinase activity is deficient.

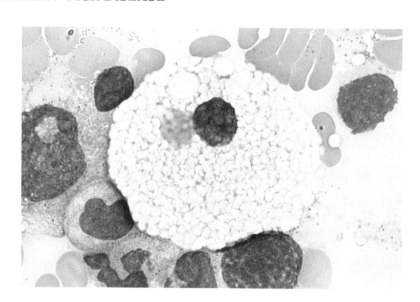

16.2. Niemann–Pick disease (type A, infantile)
Bone marrow; Sudan black for lipid

The Niemann–Pick cells stain weakly with Sudan black but may often show a red birefringence in polarized light. This figure shows the same cells viewed in polarized light (on left) and in ordinary light (on right).

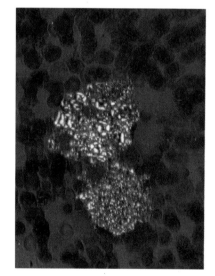 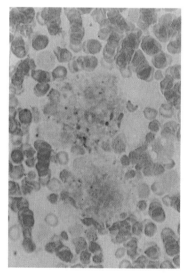

16.3. Niemann–Pick disease (type B/E adult)

Bone marrow

Abundant 'sea-blue histiocytes' are present with only a few foamy cells. These cells are packed with blue-staining granules which are also PAS-positive, Sudanophilic, and show marked autofluorescence. Unless they are numerous, and have a packed cytoplasm, the label 'sea-blue histiocyte' should not be used. The disease presents at any age from 6 months with hepatosplenomegaly but without neurological involvement. In the juvenile age range the storage cells resemble those in Niemann–Pick type A but in the older patients the 'sea-blue histiocytes' predominate.

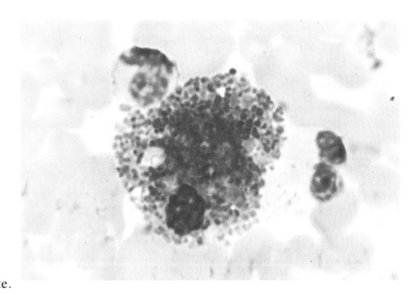

16.4. Niemann–Pick disease (type C)

Bone marrow from an infant

The numerous storage cells resemble Niemann–Pick cells but differ in having vacuoles of varying size in the same cell, and also because of the presence of densely staining nuclear debris in many cells. Occasional cells resembling sea-blue histiocytes can sometimes be found. This storage disorder may present in mid-childhood with unexplained hepatosplenomegaly. Later dementia and a defect of downward gaze appear. Many children suffer severe prolonged neonatal jaundice, without neurological deficit until mid-childhood.

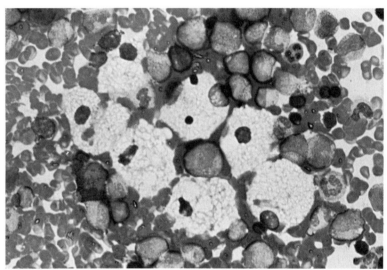

16.5. Niemann–Pick disease (type C)

Bone marrow

In the older child (and adult) the densely staining nuclear debris is more prominent than in the infant. Occasional, scattered sea-blue histiocytes (as shown in 16.3) may be formed, their numbers increasing with the age of the patient.

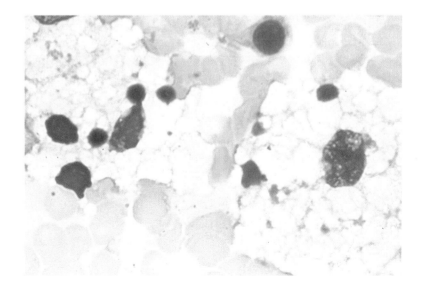

16.6. Niemann–Pick disease (type C)
Bone marrow; Sudan black (for fat)

The foam cells usually are unstained (upper right) but some may show a greyish granular cytoplasm. There is no birefringence in polarized light. The cells are PAS-positive and show strong acid phosphatase activity.

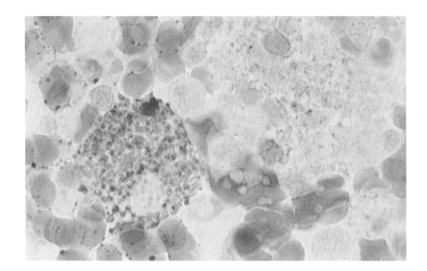

16.7. Niemann–Pick disease (type C)
Bone marrow from heterozygote

Heterozygotes also show the same foamy storage cells, but to a lesser extent. It may be difficult to distinguish carriers from the disease state and other tests are necessary.

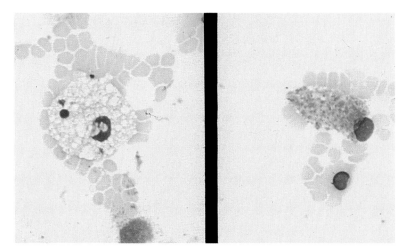

GAUCHER'S DISEASE

Infantile form: presents in infancy with marked hepatosplenomegaly, failure to thrive, and psychomotor retardation. Juvenile form: presents at age 3–4 years with hepatosplenomegaly and myoclonus. Mental retardation and a defect of horizontal gaze often also develop. Adult form: presents from 2–3 years onwards. No neurological symptoms occur. Bone pain and thrombocytopenia are common. β-Glucocerebrosidase activity is deficient.

16.8. Gaucher's disease
Bone marrow

The typical Gaucher cell has a striped appearance often likened to crumpled tissue paper, but this appearance is not always as clear as in the illustration. More cells are found in the infantile form. The Gaucher cells are sometimes multinucleate and are PAS-positive.

Foamy cells and pseudo–Gaucher cells may occur in juvenile chronic myeloid leukaemia (see 9.22 and 9.23) and in other conditions of overload of the macrophage system.

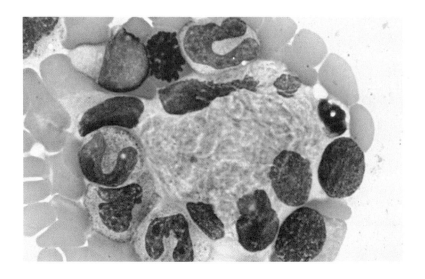

16.9. Gaucher's disease
Bone marrow; acid phosphatase stain

Gaucher cells from the infantile form, stained brown, are numerous and readily visible even at low power. Only histiocytes and storage cells show this degree of acid phosphatase activity. Megakaryocytes (only two are present) show variable low activity which is usually finely punctate.

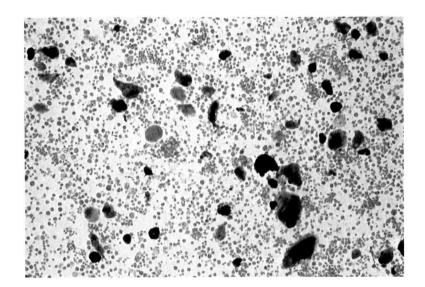

WOLMAN'S DISEASE
The infantile form presents from early infancy with hepatosplenomegaly, failure to thrive, and adrenal calcification. Death results, usually, by six months. The juvenile and adult forms (cholesteryl ester storage disease) are mild and present with mild hepatosplenomegaly. Acid esterase (acid lipase) is deficient in all forms.

16.10. Wolman's disease (and cholesteryl ester storage disease)
Blood film

Many lymphocytes contain small, well-defined cytoplasmic vacuoles. The vacuoles contain neutral fat (shown with oil red O) but since the serum is often lipaemic it can be difficult to decide whether the lipid stain is within or on the surface of the cell.

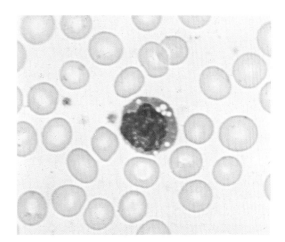

16.11. Wolman's disease (and cholesteryl ester storage disease)
Blood film; acid esterase stain

In the normal patient, acid esterase activity can be shown as a single 'block' in about 80 per cent of lymphocytes (T-lymphocytes), as shown in the right-hand picture. In Wolman's disease and cholesteryl ester storage disease, activity is found in less than 10 per cent and is less intense than normal. The left-hand picture shows a lymphocyte from a patient with Wolman's disease.

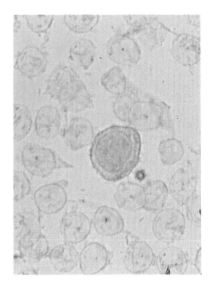
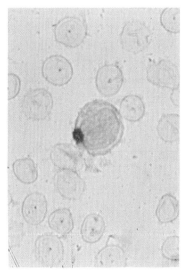

16.12. Wolman's disease
Bone marrow

Large foamy histiocytes are present and are similar to those seen in G_{M1}-gangliosidosis (see 16.19).

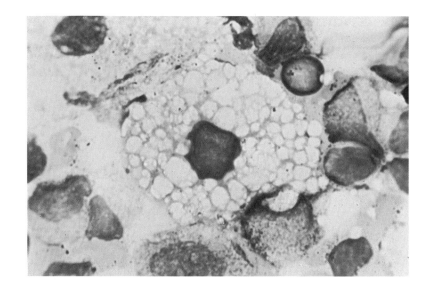

16.13. Wolman's disease
Bone marrow; oil red O for fat

The large foamy histiocytes, in contrast with other storage disorders, are filled with Sudanophilic acid. Lipid-laden histiocytes may also be seen in some hyperlipidaemias. The lipid shows birefringence in polarized light due to the presence of cholesteryl esters.

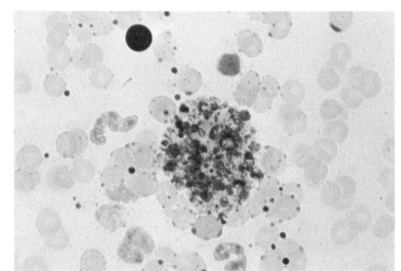

16.14. Wolman's disease
Bone marrow; Nile blue
(Cain's method)

The storage cells stain deep blue/purple indicating that free fatty acids are present in addition to the neutral fat. No other storage disease shows this reaction.

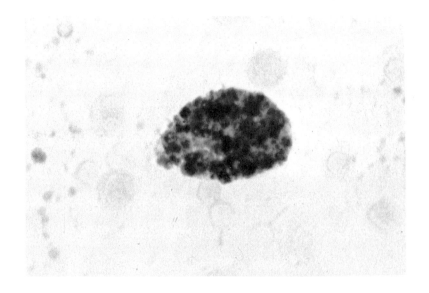

16.15. Cholesteryl ester storage disease (adult Wolman's disease)
Bone marrow

Occasional histiocytes with a few vacuoles in their cytoplasm can be found. Their appearance is not distinctive.

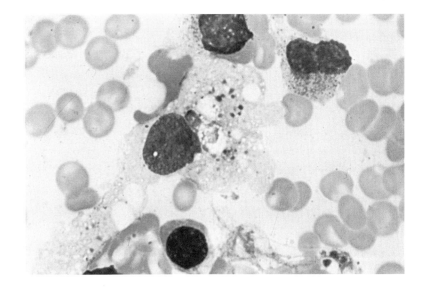

16.16. Cholesteryl ester storage disease (adult Wolman's disease)
Bone marrow; oil red O for fat

The rare histiocytes show neutral fat accumulation.

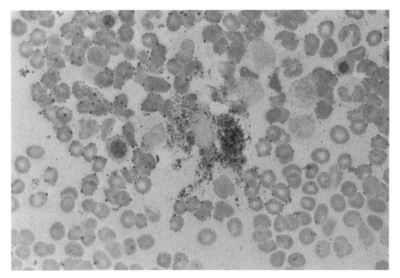

POMPE'S DISEASE
This disease presents in early infancy with hepatosplenomegaly, hypotonia, and cardiomegaly.

There are also rare juvenile forms and an adult form presenting as a muscular disorder.

Acid maltase activity is deficient.

Screening of blood films to detect lymphocytic glycogen deposits is a most reliable test, and can be also used to exclude a diagnosis of acid maltase deficiency.

16.17. Pompe's disease (glycogen storage disease II)
Blood film; PAS after celloidin protection

Small discrete vacuoles in lymphocytic cytoplasm (visible in routine MGG preparations) contain a PAS-positive, water-soluble substance—glycogen. The majority of lymphocytes are positive in the infantile form; a smaller proportion may be affected in the adult form. The glycogen content of neutrophils is normal.

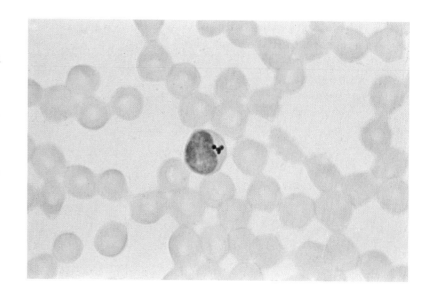

GANGLIOSIDOSIS

G_{M1}-gangliosidosis I presents in early infancy with hepatosplenomegaly, mental retardation, and skeletal deformities similar to those seen in the mucopolysaccharidoses. No mucopolysaccharides are excreted.

G_{M1}-gangliosidosis II presents in the late infantile/juvenile period, without hepatosplenomegaly or bony changes. Dementia is the main symptom.

β-galactosidase activity is deficient in both types.

16.18. G_{M1}-gangliosidosis type I
Blood film

Numerous vacuolated lymphocytes are present, more readily seen in the tail of the film. The vacuoles are multiple and larger than those of Wolman's or Pompe's disease.

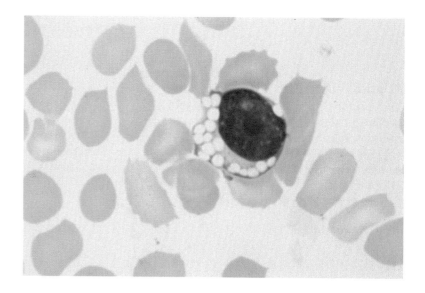

16.19. G$_{M1}$-gangliosidosis type I
Bone marrow
Numerous large foamy storage cells are found throughout the marrow. Vacuolated lymphocytes are present in the marrow film and one can be seen to the left of the storage cell.

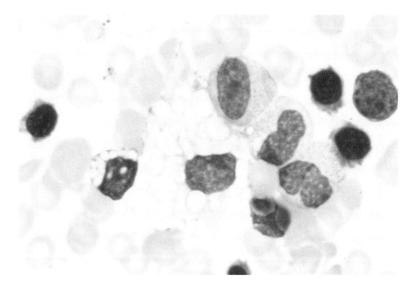

16.20. G$_{M1}$-gangliosidosis type I
Bone marrow
Other cells show cytoplasmic vacuolation. Here two eosinophil granulocytes show more vacuoles than eosinophilic granules. Peripheral blood eosinophils have fewer, larger granules many of which stain grey (see also 16.37).

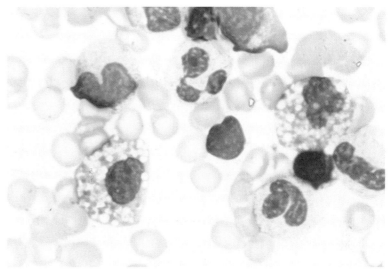

16.21. G$_{M1}$-gangliosidosis type II; late infantile
Bone marrow
Scattered storage cells with a 'sky-blue' cytoplasm can be found even when there is no splenomegaly. These cells superficially resemble Gaucher cells (see 16.6) but their characteristic blue colour distinguishes them. No vacuolated lymphocytes are seen in marrow or blood. The deficiency of β-galactosidase activity can be shown cytochemically with an indoxyl method.

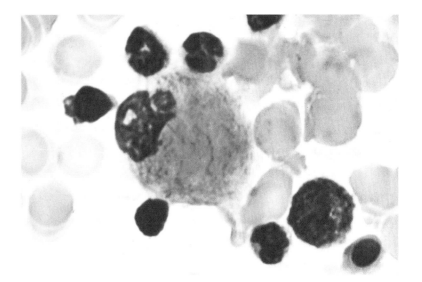

MUCOPOLYSACCHARIDOSES (MPS)

This group of conditions presents variably with skeletal deformities, coarse facies, and hepatosplenomegaly. Mental retardation is usually present. Destructive behaviour is a feature of the Sanfilippo type. Urinary mucopolysaccharides are increased in all types.

Table 16.1. The mucopolysaccharidoses

Type number	Eponym
IH	Hurler
IS	Scheie
IH/S	Hurler/Scheie compound
II	Hunter
III (A, B, C & D)	Sanfilippo
IV	Morquio, Morquio–Brailsford
VI	Maroteaux–Lamy
VII	β-glucuronidase deficiency, Sly

16.22. Mucopolysaccharidosis
Blood film

Gasser cell. These cells are lymphocytes with cytoplasmic vacuolation; purplish granules are visible within the vacuoles. The purple staining represents the remnant of mucopolysaccharide left after aqueous treatment. These cells are present in most of the mucopolysaccharidoses except Morquio's disease (MPS IV).

Vacuolated lymphocytes are not generally a feature of the MPS, although in Morquio type B (MPS IVB) the lymphocytic vacuolation may be as marked as in G_{M1}-gangliosidosis type I.

16.23. Mucopolysaccharidosis
Blood film; toluidine blue
(ref. 12)

Pink metachromatic inclusions (top of cell) are present in the lymphocytes in all types of MPS except type IV (Morquio). The proportion of lymphocytes affected is highest (> 20 per cent) in the Sanfilippo syndrome (type III), while those in patients with Hunter or Hurler syndrome show less than 20 per cent with inclusions.

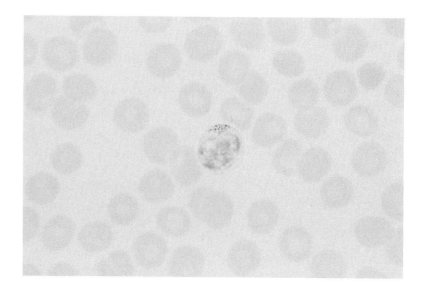

16.24. Mucopolysaccharidosis III (Sanfilippo)
Bone marrow

Few storage cells are ever seen but occasional scattered histiocytes with a stippled basophilic cytoplasm may be found. These basophilic granules are metachromatic with toluidine blue (Haust and Landing method or Muir, Mittwoch, and Bitter method (ref. 12)).

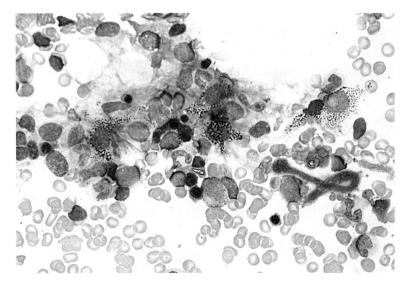

16.25. Mucopolysaccharidosis IV (Morquio)
Blood film

No metachromatic inclusions are present in MPS IV but within a proportion of neutrophils abnormal granulation can be found. The granules are often paired as in this figure.

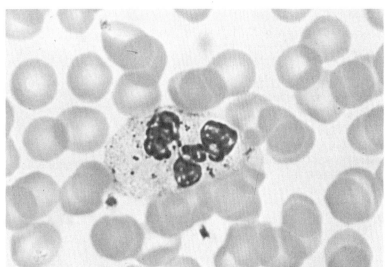

16.26. Mucopolysaccharidosis VI
Blood film

Alder granulation. All neutrophils contain this dense granulation, which resembles a rather coarse toxic granulation. It differs from toxic granulation by its metachromasia and its birefringence. Alder granulation occurs in MPS VI (Maroteaux–Lamy), in mucosulphatidosis, and also in β-glucuronidase deficiency.

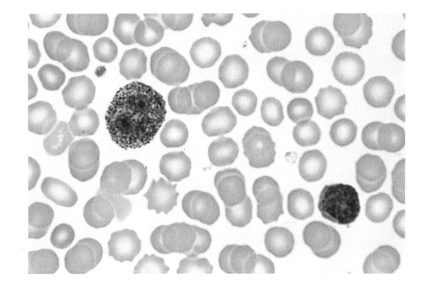

16.27. Mucopolysaccharidosis VI
Bone marrow

In MPS VI, Alder granulation is present in all granulated cells in the marrow.

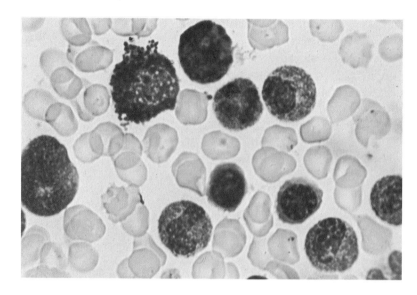

16.28. Mucopolysaccharidosis VI
Bone marrow; toluidine blue (ref. 12(b))

Apart from the metachromasia of the Alder granules, storage cells with very striking, densely-basophilic granular cytoplasm are occasionally seen in Maroteaux–Lamy syndrome (MPS VI). Although striking in appearance, these cells are not specific to MPS VI and may be seen in other MPS.

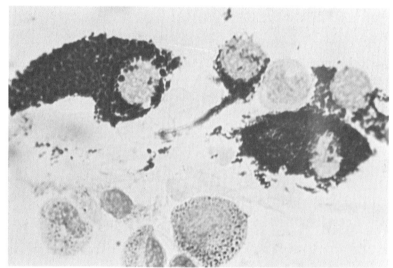

MANNOSIDOSIS

The typical presentation is of a child who appears to have one of the mucopolysaccharidoses but without mucopolysacchariduria. Mild forms also occur. The diagnosis can be confirmed by assay of WBC α-mannosidase and by the examination of the pattern of urinary oligosaccharide excretion.

16.29. Mannosidosis
Bone marrow

Numerous foamy histiocytes are present and do not stain with Sudan black. Vacuolated lymphocytes are also easily seen.

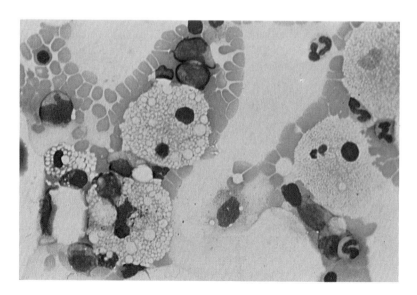

16.30. Mannosidosis
Bone marrow
Scattered plasma cells with coarse discrete vacuoles separated by strands of blue-staining cytoplasm are characteristic of mannosidosis.

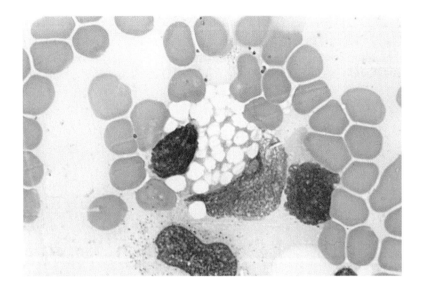

SIALIDOSIS

Sialidosis I: this condition presents in the juvenile-adolescent period with bilateral cherry-red spots at the maculae, dementia, and myoclonus. Hepatosplenomegaly is not present.

Sialidosis II (mucolipidosis I): this condition presents with the same clinical picture as a child with mucopolysaccharidosis in the infantile period. There is no mucopolysacchariduria. Neuraminidase activity is deficient.

16.31. Sialidosis I (cherry-red spot myoclonus syndrome)
Bone marrow
Foamy cells with bluish-staining vacuoles are present but are rare, and resemble odd plasma cells. They can be distinguished by their acid phosphatase activity.

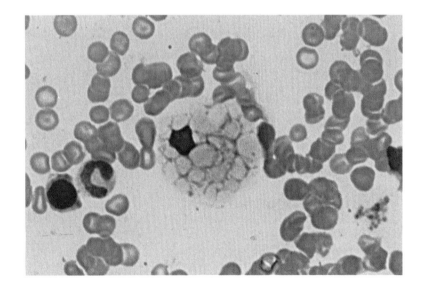

16.32. Sialidosis I
Bone marrow; PAS stain
The foamy cells, unlike any other storage cells, stain intensely with PAS.

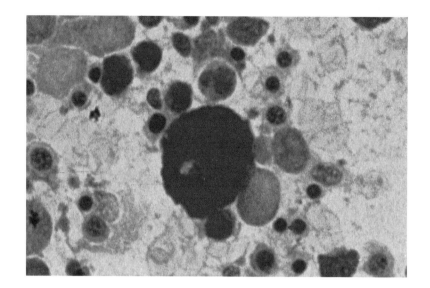

16.33. Sialidosis I
Bone marrow; acid phosphatase stain
The foamy cells show strong acid phosphatase activity (brown reaction product) at the periphery of the vacuoles. Activity in the other cells present is punctate and normal.

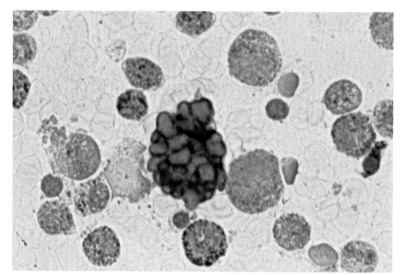

16.34. Sialidosis II (mucolipidosis I)
Blood film
A lymphocyte with many large discrete cytoplasmic vacuoles present in a blood film from a patient who presented as a mucopolysaccharidosis without mucopolysacchariduria. He had bilateral cherry-red spots at the macula and some corneal clouding. No metachromasia and no PAS-positivity can be demonstrated in these cells. Numerous cells of this type are readily visible in the 'tail' of the film and are similar to those found in I-cell disease (mucolipidosis II), G_{M1}-gangliosidosis type I, mannosidosis, juvenile Batten's disease, aspartylglucosaminuria, and the rarer sialic acid storage disease and Salla disease (see 16.18 and 16.38).

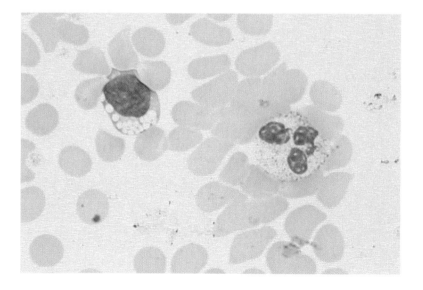

16.35. I-cell disease (mucolipidosis II)
Bone marrow

Patients with I-cell disease present as
a mucopolysaccharidosis without
mucopolysacchariduria and are usually
dwarfed. Contractures and cardiac
involvement occur during the second year.

Bone marrow generally shows little of
note except for vacuolation of some
lymphocytes (as in the peripheral blood).
Occasional osteoblasts with vacuolation
and pink inclusions may be found.

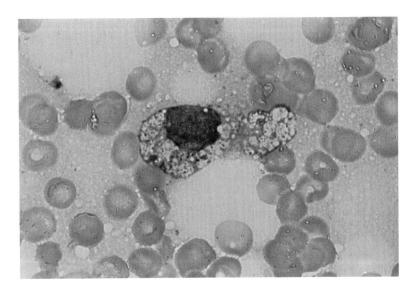

16.36. Sialic acid storage disease
Bone marrow

Large foamy storage cells with large and
small cytoplasmic vacuoles and some
erythrophagocytosis are present in this
disorder, which has clinical features of a
typical 'mucolipidosis'.

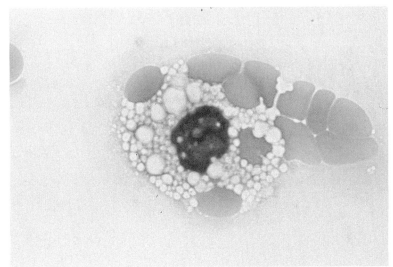

16.37. Sialic acid storage disease
Peripheral blood

Eosinophils have unusual granules that are
larger and fewer than normal, and stain
with a greyish colour. Compare the normal
eosinophil on the left with the abnormal
eosinophil on the right. Similar unusual
eosinophils are also found in G_{M1}-
gangliosidosis.

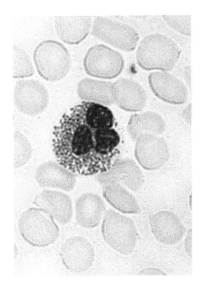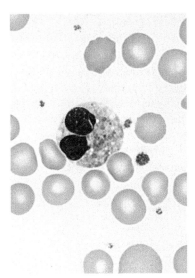

BATTEN'S DISEASE

The juvenile form presents from 5 to 8 years of age with progressive loss of vision. Dementia follows, sometimes several years later.

The late-infantile form presents at about 2 years with fits and dementia. EEG shows characteristic features.

The infantile form presents with psychomotor retardation from about 8 months of age. Microcephaly and an isoelectric EEG are later features.

16.38. Juvenile Batten's disease
Blood film

Lymphocytes, particularly in the tail of the film, show prominent coarse cytoplasmic vacuolation. Similar vacuolation is also found in I-cell disease, mannosidosis, G_{M1}-gangliosidosis I, and aspartylglucosaminuria.

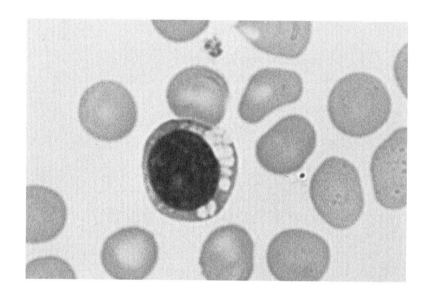

16.39. Late-infantile Batten's disease
Buffy coat preparation for electron microscopy

By light microscopy no abnormality is seen in the lymphocytic cytoplasm. By electron microscopy membrane-bound collections of curvilinear bodies are present in a high proportion of lymphocytes.

Curvilinear bodies are pathognomonic of late-infantile Batten's disease.

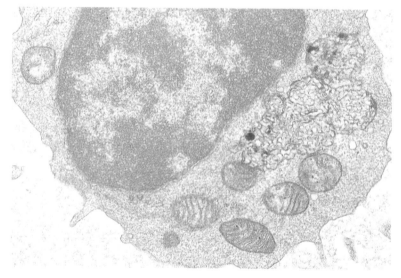

16.40. Infantile Batten's disease
Buffy coat preparation for electron microscopy

No abnormality is seen by light microscopy. By electron microscopy granular osmiophilic deposits ('GROD') are present in the cytoplasm of some lymphocytes.

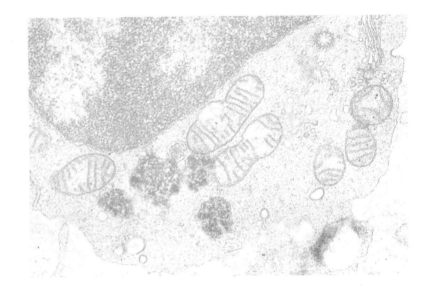

Cystinosis

Failure to thrive and the Fanconi syndrome are the presenting features. Photophobia and fair hair are also common.

16.41. Cystinosis
Bone marrow; alcoholic basic fuchsin

Histiocytes containing the water-soluble cystine crystals are best shown in *carefully* made films which have been stained in an alcoholic solution and then viewed in polarized light. The brick shaped crystals are pathognomonic. Scattered single crystals are often seen.

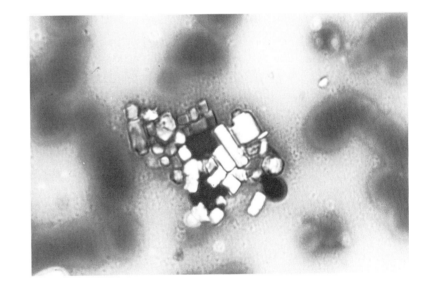

16.42. Cystinosis
Bone marrow; wet preparation

A single drop from the anticoagulated aspirate is placed on a slide, covered with a cover slip and viewed in polarized light. Numerous whole histiocytes are present containing cystine crystals with their characteristic brick shape. The hexagonal habit is not birefringent.

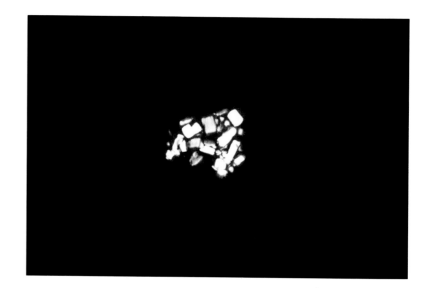

16.43. Oxalosis
Bone marrow trephine

Polarized-light. Oxalate crystals are present within the bone, but not in the marrow.

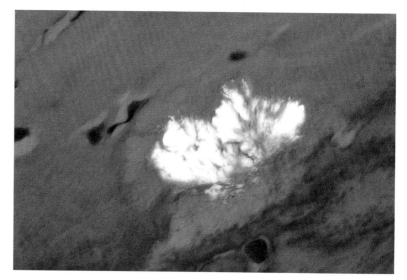

16.44. Jordans anomaly
Blood film

Neutrophils show prominent cytoplasmic vacuolation.

Jordans patients had a muscular disease that may well have been due to a carnitine deficiency or a fat oxidation defect.

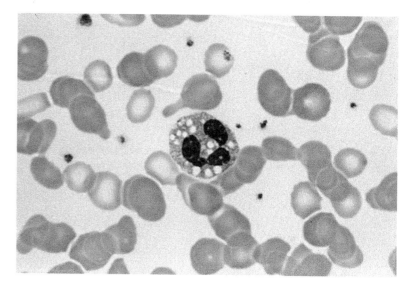

16.45. Jordans anomaly
Blood film; oil red O for fat

The prominently vacuolated neutrophils contain neutral fat which is not always readily stained. No toxic granulation is present.

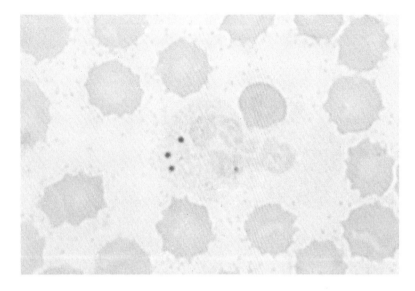

16.46. Hyperlipoproteinaemia type I
Bone marrow

Acquired 'storage' cells filled with lipid accumulate in response to the lipid overload and may be mistaken for genuine storage cells. Similar cells are found in the other forms of hyperlipidaemia.

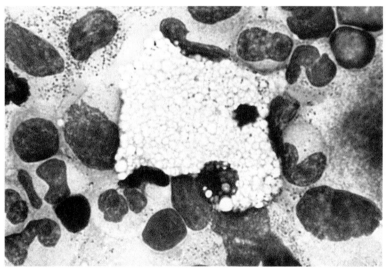

16.47. Fetal G_{M1}-gangliosidosis type I
Peripheral blood

Vacuolated lymphocytes are present in an affected 18-week-old fetus.

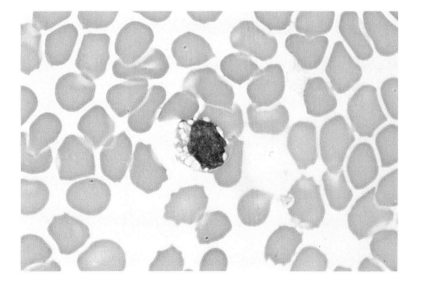

16.48. Fetal Mucopolysaccharidosis VI
Bone marrow

The storage cells are present in the marrow from at least 11 weeks gestation. Examination of bone marrow provides the quickest verification of an affected fetus terminated after biochemical detection of the disease in a chorionic villus sample. Similar cells are found in fetuses affected with mucopolysaccharidosis, and typical storage cells are found for each of the visceral storage diseases.

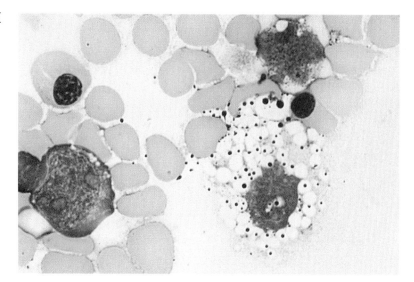

17
Artefacts

17.1. Red cell crenation
Blood film

This effect is caused by rapid drying of the blood film on a hot day.

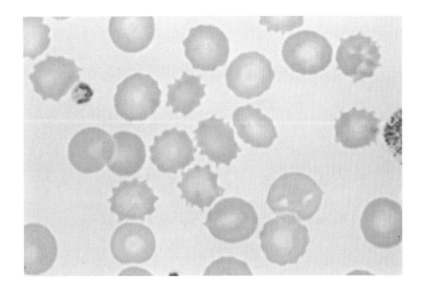

17.2. Sequestrene change
Blood film

Prolonged exposure of blood samples to sequestrene often leads to nuclear condensation in 'polymorphs' as shown here. Also seen in viraemia and septicaemia.

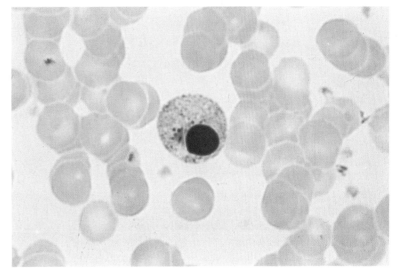

17.3. Sequestrene change
Blood film
Red cell crenation and neutrophil nuclear disintegration have occurred after sustained exposure to sequestrene.

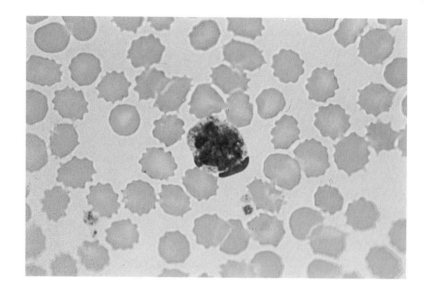

17.4. Water artefact
Blood film
Substantial water contamination of methanol fixative will produce small red cell inclusions.

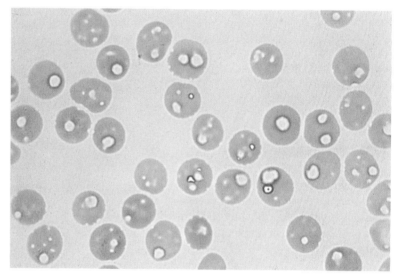

17.5. Water artefact
Blood film
In this instance, because of a high concentration of water, the inclusions have fused to form large vacuoles superficially mimicking gross hypochromia.

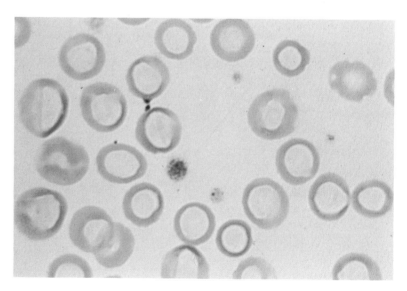

17.6. Auto-agglutination of red cells
Blood film

This child had mycoplasma pneumonia. The red cells have auto-agglutinated because they are coated with cold antibody. This agglutination occurs as the slide is dried out at room temperature and can be prevented by drying at 37°C.

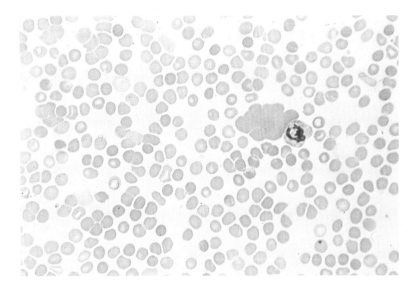

17.7. Platelet satellitism
Blood film

This artefact, in which platelets 'rosette' around polymorphs, occurs at room temperature and in some cases is due to an IgG-mediated mechanism. Lack of awareness of this phenomenon may lead to a false diagnosis of thrombocytopenia.

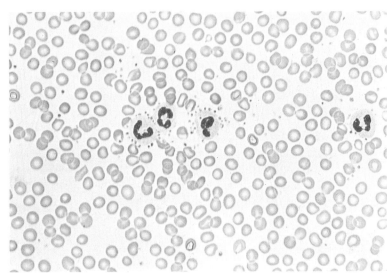

17.8. Platelet aggregation
Blood film

This effect may be seen in films made after a difficult thumb-prick procedure and must be differentiated from true thrombocytopenia.

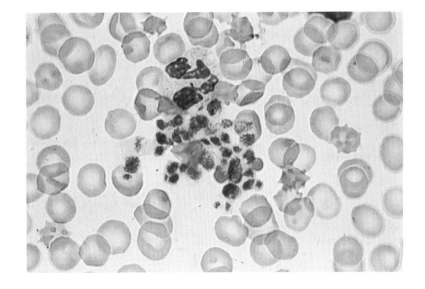

17.9. EDTA-mediated platelet clumping
Blood film

This phenomenon, due to an IgG antibody coating the platelets, causes clumping in the presence of EDTA but not other anticoagulants. It is thus another cause of 'pseudo-thrombocytopenia'.

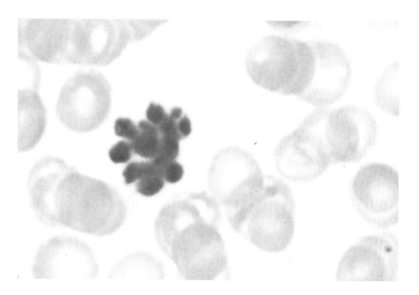

17.10. "Talc" granules
Bone marrow

Starch granules, now used instead of talc, can mimic storage cells or even parasitic infections. It usually gets on to the slides from surgical gloves.

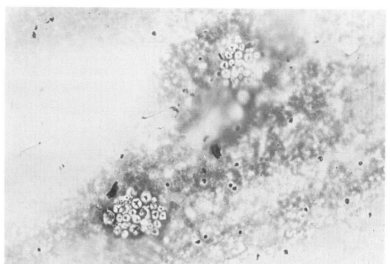

17.11. 'Pseudo-rosette'
Bone marrow

Poor spreading of marrow aspirates may lead to artificial clumps or 'rosettes', mimicking tumour infiltration, e.g. neuroblastoma.

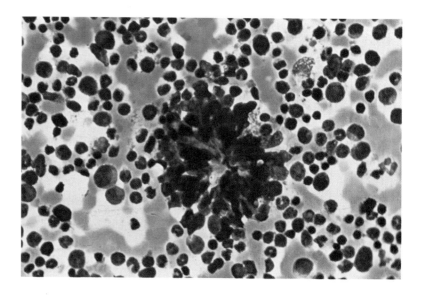

Appendix

Normal haematological values in infancy and childhood

Age	Red cell count (× 10^{12}/l)	Hb (g/dl)	PCV	MCV (fl.)	MCH (pg)	MCHC (g/dl)	Average reticulo-cytes (%)	Total WBC range (× 10^9/l)	Absolute neutrophil count (× 10^9/l)	Absolute lymphocyte count (× 10^9/l)	Absolute monocyte count (× 10^9/l)	Absolute eosinophil count (× 10^9/l)
Newborn; full term	5.1 ± 1.0	18.4 ± 2.2	0.60 ± 0.07	108 ± 9	35 ± 4	36 ± 2	3.2	9–30	4.5–13.2	2.7–11.0	0.4–3.1	0.2–0.9
7 days	5.1 ± 1.0	17.9 ± 2.5	0.56 ± 0.9	99 ± 11	32.5 ± 4	35 ± 2	0.5	5–21	1.5–10.0	2.0–17	0.3–2.7	< 0.7
3 months	4.5 ± 0.7	11.3 ± 0.5	0.33 ± 0.03	88 ± 8	29 ± 5	33 ± 3	0.7	6–15	1.5–7.0	4.0–12	0.2–1.5	< 0.7
1 year	4.5 ± 0.7	11.8 ± 0.5	0.39 ± 0.02	78 ± 8	27 ± 4	32 ± 3	0.9	6–15	1.5–7.0	5.0–10	0.2–1.5	< 0.7
3–6 years	4.5 ± 0.7	12.7 ± 1.0	0.37 ± 0.03	87 ± 8	27 ± 3	33 ± 2	1.0	5–21	2.0–6.0	5.5–8.0	0.2–1.5	< 0.7
10–12 years	4.7 ± 0.6	13.2 ± 1.0	0.39 ± 0.03	86 ± 8	27 ± 3	33 ± 2	1.0	5–21	2.0–6.0	1.5–4.0	0.2–1.5	< 0.7
Male adult	5.2 ± 0.8	16.0 ± 2.0	0.47 ± 0.05	85 ± 8	29.5 ± 2.5	33 ± 2	1.0	4.3–10	2.0–7.5	1.5–4.0	0.2–0.95	< 0.7
Female adult	4.8 ± 0.6	14.0 ± 2.0	0.42 ± 0.05	85 ± 8	29.5 ± 2.5	33 ± 2	1.0	4.3–10	2.0–7.5	1.5–4.0	0.2–0.95	< 0.7

This table is complied from several studies. Race may affect normal values; thus negroes frequently have Hbs. 0.5 g/dl lower than caucasians even after correction of iron deficiency.

Prematurity affects values, e.g. MCV of 118 fl, at 34 weeks; total WBC up to 30 per cent lower than value at term.

Abbreviations: PCV, packed cell volume; MCH, mean corpuscular haemoglobin; MCHC, mean corpuscular haemoglobin concentration; WBC, white blood cell count; MCV, mean corpuscular volume.

The Franco–American–British (FAB) classification of myelodysplastic syndromes

Class	Marrow			Peripheral blood	
	Trilineage dyshematopoiesis	Ringed sideroblasts	% Blasts	Monocytes	Blasts
Refractory anemia (RA)	+	<15%	<5	<10^9/L	<1%
Refractory anemia with sideroblasts (RA-S)	+	>15%	<5	<10^9/L	<1%
Refractory anemia with excess blasts (RAEB)	+	Any %	5–20	Any	<5%
Refractory anemia with excess blasts in transformation (RAEB-T)	+	Any %	20–30	Any	Any
Chronic myelomonocytic leukemia	+	Any %	<5	>10^9/L	—

The FAB scoring system for L1 and L2 ALL: (A zero or positive score = L1; A negative score = L2)

Criteria*	Score†
High N/C ratio ≥75% of cells	+
Low N/C ratio ≥25% of cells	−
Nucleoli: 0 to 1 (small) ≥75% of cells	+
Nucleoli: 1 or more (prominent) ≥25% of cells	−
Irregular nuclear membrane ≥25% of cells	−
Large cells ≥50% of cells	−

* The following are not scored: (1) intermediate or indeterminate criteria, (2) regular nuclear membrane in ≥75% of cells, and (3) <50% large cells, regardless of cell size heterogeneity.

† Positive (+), or negative (−).

Revised criteria for the classification of AML

Bennett, J.A., et al. (1985) *Annals of Internal Medicine* **103**, 626–629.

M₁

1. Blast cells, agranular and granular types (types I and II) more than 90 per cent of non-erythroid cells. At least 3 per cent of these peroxidase or Sudan Black-positive.
2. Remaining 10 per cent of cells (or less) are maturing granulocytes or monocytes.

M₂

1. Sum of agranular and granular blasts (types I and II) is from 30 to 89 per cent of non-erythroid cells.
2. Monocytic cells, less than 20 per cent.
3. Granulocytes from promyelocytes to mature polymorphs, more than 10 per cent.

M₃

1. Majority of cells are abnormal promyelocytes with heavy granulation.
2. Characteristic cells containing bundles of Auer rods ('faggots') invariably present.

M₄

1. In the marrow, blasts more than 30 per cent of non-erythroid cells.
2. Sum of myeloblasts, promyelocytes, myelocytes and later granulocytes is between 30 and 80 per cent of non-erythroid cells.
3. More than 20 per cent of non-erythroid cells are monocyte lineage.
4. If monocytic cells exceed 80 per cent, diagnosis is M_5.

   Note
   (a) If marrow findings as above and peripheral blood monocytes (all types) are more than $5.0 \times 10^9/l$, diagnosis is M_4.
   (b) If monocyte count less than $5.0 \times 10^9/l$, M_4 can be confirmed on basis of serum lysozyme, combined esterase, etc.
   (c) Diagnosis of M_4 confirmed if more than 20 per cent of marrow precursors are monocytes (confirmed by special stains).

M₄ with eosinophilia

1. Eosinophils more than 5 per cent of non-erythroid cells in marrow.
2. Eosinophils are abnormal.
3. Eosinophils are chloroacetate- and PAS-positive.

M₅

1. 80 per cent or more of marrow non-erythroid cells are monoblasts, promonocytes or monocytes.
2. M_5a, 80 per cent of monocytic cells are monoblasts.
3. M_5b, less than 80 per cent of monocytic cells are monoblasts, remainder are predominantly promonocytes and monocytes.

M₆

1. The erythroid component of the marrow exceeds 50 per cent of all nucleated cells.
2. 30 per cent or more of the remaining non-erythroid cells are agranular or granular blasts (types I and II).

   Note: if more than 50 per cent erythroid cells but less than 30 per cent blasts, diagnosis becomes myelodysplastic syndrome.

M₇

1. 30 per cent at least of nucleated cells are blasts.
2. Blasts identified by platelet peroxidase on EM, or by monoclonal antibodies.
3. Increased reticulin is common.

References

Staining methods

1. Acid esterase: Lake, B. D. (1971). *J. clin. Path.* **24**, 617.
2. Acid phosphatase: (a) Lake, B. D. *Jl R. microsc. Soc.* **85**, 73.
   (b) Goldberg, A. F. (1962). *Nature, Lond.* **195**, 197.
3. Esterase, non-specific and chloro-acetate: Yam, L. T., Li, C. Y., and Crosby, W. H. (1971). *Am. J. clin. Path.* **55**, 283.
4. Iron stain: Douglas, A. S. and David, J. C. (1953). *J. clin. Path.* **6**, 307.
5. Kleihauer stain (Hb F): Neinhaus, K. and Betke, K. (1968). *Klin. Wschr.* **46**, 47.
6. Neutrophil alkaline phosphatase: Hayhoe, F. G. H., Quaglino, D., and Doll, R. (1969). *Cytology and Cytochemistry of the Acute Leukaemias.* H.M.S.O., London.
7. Nile-blue: Cain, A. J. (1947). *Q. Jl microsc. Sci.* **88**, 467.
8. Nitro-blue tetrazolium: Park, B. H. and Good, R. A. (1970). *Lancet* **2**, 616.
9. Periodic acid Schiff (PAS): (a) Lake, B. D. (1970). *Histochem. J.* **2**, 441.
   (b) McManus, J. F. A. (1966). *Nature, Lond.* **158**, 202.
10. Peroxidase: Osgood, E. E. and Ashworth, C. M. (1937). *Atlas of Haematology;* Pub. J. W. Stacey, San Francisco quoted in Wintrobe, M. M. (1961). *Clinical haematology.* M. Kimpton, Philadelphia.
11. Sudan black: Lison's method quoted in Sandoz (1952) *Atlas of Haematology.* Basle.
12. Toluidine Blue: (a) Muir, H., Mittwoch, U., and Bitter, T. (1963). *Archs Dis. Childh.* **38**, 358.
    (b) Haust, D. and Landing, B. H. (1961). *J. Histochem. Cytochem.* **9**, 79.

General

13. *Blood and its disorders:* Hardisty, R. M. and Weatherall, D. J. Pub. Blackwell, Oxford (2nd edition 1982.)
14. *Haematologic problems in the newborn:* Oski, F. A., Naiman, J. L. (1972). Pub. W. B. Saunders Co., Philadelphia.
15. *Haematology:* Williams, W. J., Beutler, E., Erslev, E. J., and Rundles, R. W. (1977). Pub. McGraw-Hill, New York.
16. *Haematology of infancy and childhood* (3rd edn): Nathan, D. G. and Oski, F. A. (1988). Pub. W. B. Saunders Co., London and Toronto.
17. *Lysosomes and storage diseases:* Hers, H. G. and Van Hoof, F. (ed.) (1973). Pub. Academic Press, New York, London.
18. *Practical haematology* (5th edn): Dacie, J. V. and Lewis S. M. (1975) Pub. Churchill Livingstone, Edinburgh.
19. *Proposals for classification of the acute leukaemias:* French—American—British (FAB) Co-operative Group; Bennett, J. M., Catovsky, D., Daniel, M. T. *et al.* (1976, 1981). *Br. J. Haemat.* **33**, 451 and **47**, 553.
20. *Smith's blood diseases of infancy and childhood* (4th edn): Miller, D. R., Pearson, H. A., Baehner, R. L., and McMillan, C. W. (1978). Pub. C. V. Mosby, St. Louis.
21. *Diseases of children in the subtropics and tropics.* Jelliffe, D. B. and Paget Stanfield, J. (ed.) (1978). Pub. Arnold, London.

Index